Identifying
Postural
Imbalances
Through Yoga

Identifying
Postural
Imbalances
Through Yoga

An Innovative Guide to Yoga Asana Observation and Adjustment for Your Postural Type

Revised Edition

Vayu Jung Doohwa

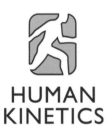

**HUMAN
KINETICS**

First published in 2019. This revised edition published in 2024 by
Lotus Publishing
Apple Tree Cottage, Inlands Road, Nutbourne, Chichester, PO18 8RJ, and
Human Kinetics
1607 N. Market Street, Champaign, Illinois 61820

United States and International
Website: **US.HumanKinetics.com**
Email: info@hkusa.com
Phone: 1-800-747-4457

Canada
Website: **Canada.HumanKinetics.com**
Email: info@hkcanada.com

Illustrations Jeon Ho Yun
Photographs Kim Mu Geon
Text Design Medlar Publishing Solutions Pvt Ltd., India
Cover Design Chris Fulcher
Printed and Bound Replika Press Pvt Ltd., India

Medical Disclaimer
This publication is written and published to provide accurate and authoritative information relevant to the subject matter presented. It is published and sold with the understanding that the author and publishers are not engaged in rendering legal, medical, or other professional services by reason of their authorship or publication of this work. If medical or other expert assistance is required, the services of a competent professional person should be sought.

British Library Cataloging-in-Publication Data
A CIP record for this book is available from the British Library

Library of Congress Cataloging-in-Publication Data
Names: Doohwa, Vayu Jung, 1968- author.
Title: Identifying postural imbalances through yoga / Vayu Jung Doohwa.
Description: Revised edition. | Champaign : Human Kinetics, 2024. |
    Includes index.
Identifiers: LCCN 2023016092 (print) | LCCN 2023016093 (ebook) |
    ISBN 9781718226982 (paperback) | ISBN 9781718226999 (epub) |
    ISBN 9781718227002 (pdf)
Subjects: LCSH: Hatha yoga. | Posture. | BISAC: HEALTH & FITNESS / Yoga |
    MEDICAL / Sports Medicine
Classification: LCC RA781.7 .D67 2024 (print) | LCC RA781.7 (ebook) |
    DDC 615.8/24--dc23/eng/20230502
LC record available at https://lccn.loc.gov/2023016092
LC ebook record available at https://lccn.loc.gov/2023016093

ISBN: 978-1-7182-2698-2
10 9 8 7 6 5 4 3 2 1

Contents

Foreword

In the tradition of Ashtanga Vinyasa Yoga, Guruji (Shri K Pattabhi Jois) would say, "99% practice, 1% theory." If this sutra is taken too literally, the student of Ashtanga Vinyasa Yoga can fall into a trap…

"The ordinary thinking mind" (that part of our thinking process that is not really awake, trapped in the cycles of conditioned thinking) will simply add 99% and 1% to get 100%. This is incorrect math, for you cannot add together two different items; for example, if you had 99 bananas and 1 apple and add these items together—yes, you arrive at 100 fruits, but you still only have 99 bananas and 1 apple.

When I met Vayu in 2008 in Beijing, China, he was teaching Yoga Anatomy on a Teacher Training Course, and I was visiting China to share in the teachings of Guruji. Vayu, I could tell, had a very sharp and intelligent mind, but I could also see that he was teaching from that "ordinary" place—teaching the same way it has always been taught, because "that is how it has always been done."

The alchemy between us, however, was tangible and we were instantly caught deep in discussion. Vayu's eyes lit up and his mind began to shine. This meeting was the beginning of a work/practice/research/inquiry partnership that is still blossoming today…

Contemporary yoga and yoga anatomy are very alive, still rooted in tradition, but now that most of the great gurus have passed to the afterworld, it is time for INNOVATION!

When like-minded people come together, innovation blossoms; in this book, you will discover that Vayu has taken many 1% theories and practiced 99% on the mat, and in his teaching has revealed some extraordinary gems. This book is pure innovation and will serve the yoga community well. I have been looking forward to seeing this edition printed in English, for this work needs to circulate around the global yoga community.

"Posture, free breathing, looking place" is another favorite of Guruji's sutras. Here, Guruji gives the student of Ashtanga Vinyasa Yoga a very simple 1% theory, but it is very difficult to achieve. What Guruji is teaching here is that correct posture sets the conditions for balanced breathing, and together balanced posture and breathing set the conditions to be able to see all and receive all from the heart sukha or "looking place."

If you look around in public places, what you will see is ordinary or poor posture reflecting that, as the Buddha once said, "there is suffering" (Dukkha). Life has many challenges and traumas for us all, and every bump, fall, or emotional trauma is stored in our bodies. You could say we are a collection of compensations held in the body.

Yoga asana, if understood and practiced correctly, is a remedy for releasing these held postural patterns. Within this book, Vayu gives the perfect tools for the student to identify and work through their own patterns. The text shows the student what to observe and how to adjust for the imbalances held within ordinary posture, along with instructions on how to breathe in a clear and simple way; this all leads to the "posture of eclipse," a neutral self-supporting spine, awakening the Sushumna and allowing the students to see all from the heart.

"Ashtanga Vinyasa Yoga Scientific Method"—Vayu has taken this sutra of Guruji to heart, and in his own practice has reflected and allowed himself to be the scientist that he is and to innovate. He has really looked into what was happening with him in his own body, and so scientifically put his own body-breath-mind into experimentation to discover himself as a typical P (posterior) body type. Vayu shared his insights during our last JSY CPD in January 2016 in London, where, as a 500-hour graduate, he presented a class called "Yoga Adjustment According to Postural Types A, P, C." The results within the practice group were astounding and enlightening. This book is the conclusion of Vayu's work and passion for inquiry. Fantastic work, Vayu! You are certainly an extraordinary man and yogi…

John Scott, 2018

Acknowledgments

I would first of all like to extend my sincere gratitude to my family, friends, students, and colleagues who have encouraged me to write this book and helped me on this journey.

A special thanks to John Scott for his love and devoted teaching. In 2008 John planted the seeds of yoga in me, and to this day he keeps on inspiring and supporting my practice and teaching. Meeting John and studying with him made me realize my own imbalances; this was the beginning of an understanding of the imbalances of others and the ways to heal them.

My wholehearted gratitude to my friend Irina Pashkevich Bourdier, who was my patient collaborator in producing the English version of this book. She has been a driving force in translating, editing, and finding a great publisher. Without Irina, the English edition of this book would never have seen the light of day.

My thanks also:

to Jon Hutchings for taking on the job of publishing this English edition;

to Jeon Ho Yun for designing and producing all the drawings with passion, perfection, and patience;

to Kim Mu Geon for the professional and beautiful photography;

to Arjuna, Kim Eun Ha, Lee Young Jin, and Jung Min Joo for bravely modeling the postural types;

to Caroline Abbot and Moira Purves for proofreading our last draft and providing valuable feedback;

and to all the students who have ever practiced with me, as well as to those who took part in the practical yoga anatomy workshops, keeping an open mind and helping me devise the concepts presented in this book.

For their love and dedication, my heartfelt gratitude to my wife, Min Jeong, and my daughter, Lia, who always greet me with a genuine smile.

Last, but not least, my deepest gratitude to my father and mother. No language has the capacity to express my love and respect for them.

This book goes out to the world thanks to the participation of many people. Whenever I contemplate gratitude, I realize that we are all connected through the Great Heart of all.

Peace…

Vayu Jung Doohwa
December 2018

Namaste
I hope this book will shed a gentle light on your yoga journey, so that the wisdom within can help you find your true self.

Introduction

How to Observe, Align, and Adjust Postural Imbalances on the Basis of Postural Type

This book is for yoga practitioners of all levels. It begins with the "know-how" and fundamentals of postural imbalances and guides you through the observation and adjustment of these imbalances, on the basis of the postural type of the practitioner. I have tried to avoid complex anatomical references and opted instead to use simple diagrams and images. These visual aids make it easier to convey my ideas more clearly. I also hope they are simple for teachers and practitioners to follow during self-experimentation.

Just as a doctor would prescribe the most relevant treatment after a thorough examination and diagnosis, you will be able to recognize unbalanced postural patterns through observation, and "prescribe" the most appropriate alignments or adjustments. Understanding postural types will guide you toward the correct adjustments in order to restore balance to your body.

In Part I of this book, I explain how to observe imbalances. In Part II, you will learn postural types systemically according to section imbalance patterns. In Part III, I recommend specific ways and principles of adjustment for the different postural types.

The Path of Yoga

Yoga is the path toward true happiness, beyond the restless mind. This journey to our middle path in life is reached through a multitude of yoga practices. One of these is called *asana* in Sanskrit. The original meaning of this term is simply to sit still for meditation. This is a challenging task for most of us, because of various bodily imbalances. Consequently, to arrive at the balanced sitting pose, yogis developed different types of poses. The aim is to restore the equilibrium of the body, leading to healthy breathing patterns, a balanced mind, and a stable seated asana.

What if You Cannot Perform a Certain Pose or a Certain Group of Poses?

It is incredibly rare for people to perform every yoga asana perfectly well. If someone can do a certain pose relatively well, they might still have difficulty performing some other poses. It is common for practitioners to have problems with asanas which are weighted toward a particular direction. For example, if a student finds that forward bends are easy, they will most probably find backward bends difficult. Similarly, if right-side poses are easy, left-side poses might be challenging. An inclination toward one or other pattern of imbalance in yoga asana practice is a manifestation of our daily life imbalances.

It is well known that in professional sport, players develop their more dominant side. Whether right or left is their preference, this is intentionally developed to compete successfully.

When it comes to practicing yoga asanas, the aim lies in restoring balance. Thus, rather than reinforcing those asanas which are already easy and strong for us, we should aim to learn and befriend the challenging ones. This is the purpose of yoga asana practice.

When we work on our weaker asanas or take our less natural direction, we struggle. Our breathing becomes heavy and pain comes, almost forcing us to give up the challenge… and we tend to avoid it. We may feel that our naturally easy asana deepens and think that our practice is progressing; however, the weak asana in fact becomes a shadow, a phantom. It is unseen, unfelt, but nevertheless it is always there.

On the other hand, forceful practice of the difficult poses often causes injuries. If we keep on using force, we only develop new, destructive patterns. Consequently, despite the long-term efforts, we do not improve our weak poses or directions, and often severe body imbalances come to the surface.

Beginners, advanced practitioners, and teachers often wonder about ways to deal with the imbalances of the body and weighted/preferential poses or directions. I believe that all yoga asana practitioners would benefit greatly from acquiring a genuine awareness of this subject. Developing a sharp eye for an unbalanced pose and a change of perspective is a good path toward approaching a general equilibrium.

Unbalanced Patterns Recognized in Yoga Poses

Imbalances in the human body can be easily recognized in yoga poses. If you can correctly distinguish the basic area of a body imbalance and its cause, you will be able to design a yoga asana path to return to the neutral state. Fortunately, there is an order in the imbalance patterns and this will help you to recognize these patterns and eliminate them.

Postural imbalance is based on musculoskeletal imbalance. The musculoskeletal system consists of bones, as well as the muscular and nervous systems. The voluntary nervous system controls voluntary movement of the muscles, which in turn move the bones. Thus, it is theoretically feasible to improve the musculoskeletal imbalance with our determination and active effort.

As a result of our long-term habitual behaviors, however, the spine and pelvic muscles become set and fixed, making change very challenging. After years of forming bodily imbalance, a long period of time is required to correct it, assuming the cause is accurately identified. In order to find the balance, I would recommend, first, to do your self-practice consistently for a long period of time. Subsequently, you should invest time in learning the theory of yoga asana, so that you can better understand the patterns of your own imbalance.

There is no need to master every theoretical aspect of yoga. A lot will be gradually revealed and healed through your self-practice and your direct experience, which is a cornerstone of yoga.

Movements and postures of the human body are affected by contractions of the muscles, and so an understanding of their actions is essential. However, this does not mean that you can only start practicing yoga once you have studied over 400 sets of muscles; you can begin with a simple awareness of the unbalanced sections and lines of the body, which are connected with the muscles.

A good analogy would be that when you take an underground train, you do not need to know every single station: the departure point and the arrival station of the line you need to take are sufficient. Over time, when you repeat the same journey, you learn to recognize other stations. The same principle applies to understanding the major body lines.

Our muscles act by connecting with the front, back, and sides of the human body as an integral line, rather than as individual, separate muscles, as often described in anatomy books. There is no need to think too scrupulously about the muscles' lines. When you bend forward or backward, you feel that the back or front side of your body stretches; this is a good enough starting point.

Basic Terms Used in This Book

In forward bends, the back side of the body is lengthened because of the contraction of the muscles of the front side. We can call the whole structure of the stretched back muscles linked to the muscle fascia the *back line*.

In backward bends, the front side of the body is lengthened because of the contraction of the muscles of the back side. Consequently, the structure of the lengthened front side of the body can be further regarded as the *front line*.

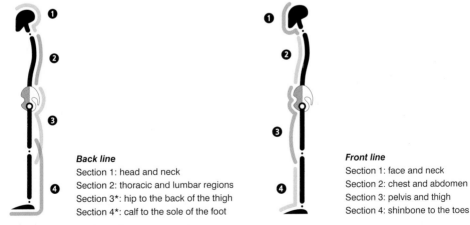

Back line
Section 1: head and neck
Section 2: thoracic and lumbar regions
Section 3*: hip to the back of the thigh
Section 4*: calf to the sole of the foot

Front line
Section 1: face and neck
Section 2: chest and abdomen
Section 3: pelvis and thigh
Section 4: shinbone to the toes

Figure I.1. *Back and front lines.*
*Sections 3 and 4 (muscles of the backs of the legs and muscles of the calves respectively) intersect each other.

For the efficient observation of the imbalances of the front and back lines, we can think of dividing each line into several sections.

Figure I.1 demonstrates how to begin to observe postural imbalances by dividing the back and front sides of the body into several sections in relation to the joints; we will refer to this as a *functional unit*.

If a practitioner finds it relatively easy to perform a forward bend, but a backward bend is challenging, as depicted in the left image of Figure I.2, this would indicate that the back line can be lengthened relatively easily. In contrast, the front line, illustrated in the right image of Figure I.2, is probably tight, which signifies a relative body imbalance.

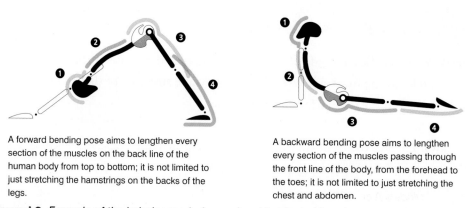

A forward bending pose aims to lengthen every section of the muscles on the back line of the human body from top to bottom; it is not limited to just stretching the hamstrings on the backs of the legs.

A backward bending pose aims to lengthen every section of the muscles passing through the front line of the body, from the forehead to the toes; it is not limited to just stretching the chest and abdomen.

Figure I.2. *Example of the imbalances in forward and backward bends.*

In the case of Figure I.2, the appropriate approach to a balanced correction would be to continuously work on lengthening the front line that is not easily stretched. This may sound like a very simple problem-solving technique—and it is. However, experience shows that even once we are able to bend forward in one pose with ease, we may still struggle to bend forward in another pose. **The key to understanding a complex imbalance is to observe the practitioner in various poses and to then compare the imbalances of the sections**.

If you start to observe the body in terms of the sections, and how they relate to each other, you will learn to recognize the patterns of individual imbalances. Let us have a quick look into one of the major concepts of this book and experiment with your own body in an upright position.

If you lift your tailbone (anterior pelvic tilt), you will find that Section 2 of the back line shortens, whereas if you drop your tailbone (posterior pelvic tilt), Section 2 of the back line lengthens. In contrast, in the case of Section 3, if you lift your tailbone, your Section 3 lengthens, and if you drop your tailbone, you will feel Section 3 shortening.

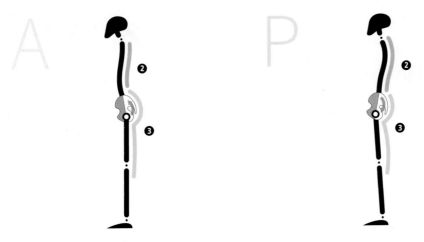

Figure I.3. *Models A and P indicating anterior and posterior pelvic tilt body types.*

Figure I.3 depicts two models, A and P. Let us assume that these are their regular standing postures. Looking at these postural patterns would lead us to suspect imbalances of the part of the Sections 2 and 3 from the lumbar region to the pelvis. In real life, though, we are not likely to come across severe imbalances, which are quickly and easily observed in a standing position. This is especially true in the yoga world, where we know how to "hide" an unbalanced pattern through either raising the tailbone or lowering it in Mountain pose (Tadasana or Samasthiti) in order to lengthen or shorten Sections 2 or 3.

On the other hand, when it comes to other, more complex, yoga poses, it is much harder to hide an imbalance. For example, one may strain to lift or drop their tailbone because of a mounting pressure between Sections 1 and 4 in a forward or backward bend. An unbalanced pattern of a pose then becomes exposed to clear observation, and the only option is to face and solve this problem.

Another fairly typical example is illustrated by the A and P models in Figure I.4. In this case, when in Downward-facing dog pose (Adho Mukha Svanasana) practitioners cannot tilt their pelvis, which is fixed posteriorly or anteriorly.

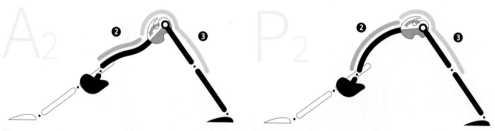

Figure I.4. *Imbalances of A and P models in Downward-facing dog pose.*

Model A in Figure I.4 shows an imbalance where Section 2 is shortened and Section 3 is consequently elongated, with the tailbone lifted. Model P demonstrates an unbalanced pattern in Section 2, which is overly elongated, and Section 3 is shortened with a dropped tailbone.

You can observe how these unbalanced patterns in Sections 2 and 3 are repeated in different poses, for example the Staff pose (Dandasana) as illustrated in Figure I.5 by A and P models.

This inequality between Sections 2 and 3 represents an imbalance in the lumbar and hip joints, which would indicate that the lumbar joints or hip joints of connective tissues are mobile in one direction but limited in the opposite direction. The key to solving the puzzle of an imbalance will be to examine which joint and which direction cause the problem. Part I of this book will explore what to observe and how to observe it in various yoga poses.

This book advocates the concept of four postural types, which are used to facilitate an understanding of the postural imbalances, particularly Sections 2 and 3 as the center

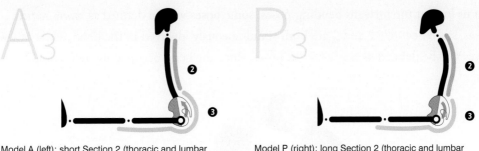

Model A (left): short Section 2 (thoracic and lumbar regions) and long Section 3 (hip and back of the leg).

Model P (right): long Section 2 (thoracic and lumbar regions) and short Section 3 (hip and back of the leg).

Figure I.5. *Imbalances of A and P models in Staff pose.*

of the body. A *postural type* is defined on the basis of the **curvature of the spine, pelvis inclination, and breathing pattern**. This will be explained in Part II of the book.

The postural type provides a criterion for the straightforward identification and classification of the patterns of imbalance. Once you understand the workings of the postural type system, you can develop your awareness of an imbalance direction in a given joint, and the principles of alignment and adjustment will become intuitive. If you learn to stretch a muscle within a shortened section and strengthen a muscle in the elongated or weaker section, this will open the pathway to a more balanced body. Moreover, the intention of the adjustment will become increasingly transparent, and your own practice and your body will become more neutral and balanced.

Why There Can Be Conflicting Adjustments for the Same Pose

Over the past 10 years, I have given presentations at many practical yoga anatomy workshops, and have seen many yogis and yoga teachers confused and asking questions such as:

Q1: Should I lift the tailbone up or drop it down in forward bends?

Q2: Should I rotate the hip joints externally or internally in Downward-facing dog?

Q3: Should I contract the gluteus maximus or relax it in Upward-facing dog pose?

The answer is, it all depends on the pose and the postural type.

Let us look at the forward bending poses: some poses will be defined as *multi-section* poses, since Sections 2 and 3 are both simultaneously involved in the bend, while other poses will be defined as *single-section* poses, since the bend occurs only in Section 2.

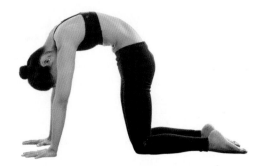

Figure I.6. *Cat pose (Marjaryasana).*

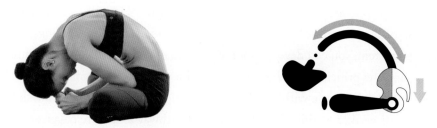

Figure I.7. *Bound angle pose (Baddha Konasana B).*

On the one hand, in the case of single-section poses, such as a Cat pose (Marjaryasana) or a Bound angle pose B (Baddha Konasana B), we only need to bend Section 2 through the action of bringing the tailbone down, regardless of the postural type.

On the other hand, in the case of a multi-section pose, such as a Seated forward bend (Paschimottanasana), the goal of the adjustment might be different, and the adjustment should be made according to the postural type.

For postural Type A, the tailbone should be guided downward, i.e., a posterior pelvic tilt, so that the shortened Section 2 (back line) of this postural type can be lengthened.

The adjustment for Type P would be the opposite—the tailbone should be guided upward (anterior pelvic tilt). You can even add a slight bend in the knees to enable a

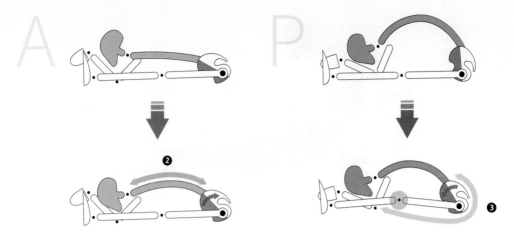

Figure I.8. *Postural Types A and P and respective imbalances.*

deeper stretch of the shortened Section 3 of the back line. Such movements promote a balance between Sections 2 and 3—the lumbar region and the hip joint (Figure I.8). A more definitive, step-by-step, approach, with tools and Q&As for postural Types A and P are presented in Part III of this book.

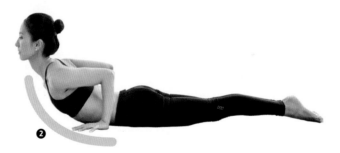

Figure I.9. *Cobra pose (Bhujangasana)—a single-section backward bending pose, only lengthening Section 2.*

The method for backward bending is similar: we have single-section poses, which only lengthen Section 2, and multi-section poses, which lengthen both Sections 2 and 3. For example, Cobra (Figure I.9) is a single-section pose, which only lengthens Section 2 of the front line.

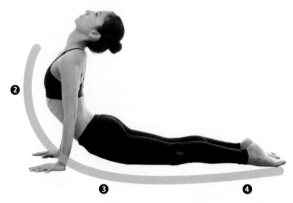

Figure I.10. *Upward-facing dog pose (Urdhva Mukha Svanasana)—a multi-section pose, lengthening simultaneously Sections 2 and 3.*

An alternative example is Upward-facing dog pose (Urdhva Mukha Svanasana); this is a multi-section backward bending pose, in which both Sections 2 and 3 of the front line lengthen together (Figure I.10).

The majority of backward bending poses are multi-sectional, and we should aim to lengthen Sections 2 and 3 simultaneously.

By following this logic, forward and backward bending poses could be adjusted differently, depending on the type of pose and postural type. Understanding this methodology is a helpful tool in observing and following clearly an intended adjustment.

In this book, I attempt to provide simple and systematic answers to many questions like the ones mentioned above, which yoga practitioners and teachers are so eager to understand.

In Parts I and II, you will learn how to identify your own postural type, through observation and classification. In Part III you will learn the definitive principles and methods of step-by-step adjustments.

My teacher, John Scott, planted the seed of the Ashtanga Vinyasa Yoga tradition within me. In the last 10 years I have been practicing and exploring yoga with my students in the daily teacher-assisted self-practice classes. Most of the ideas in this book have therefore come from my direct experience. Furthermore, this kind of experiential observation and classification of the postural types and adjustment methods is obviously a relative tool, not an absolute formula. We can align and adjust better with knowledge of the postural type methodology.

"We see the world as it is when our mind is at peace. When it is not, we see merely what we want to see."

PART I

OBSERVATION

   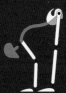

1
Recognizing Patterns of Imbalance

● ● ● ● ● ●

As mentioned in the Introduction, imbalances in the body can be identified through yoga asana practice. Asanas, or poses, are an excellent medium for both discovering and correcting these imbalances.

Generally speaking, body imbalances would be diagnosed by specialists; however, instead of being overly dependent on posture assessment tests, many yoga practitioners and teachers believe that self-assessment of their own imbalances through asanas is a preferable and more effective option. This is because imbalances in the human body are not something that can be corrected within a short period of time: they are a lifelong condition that will gradually improve through long-term, regular management. With perseverance, you will see results over time.

In addition, postural imbalances are usually identified through assessment methods, using equipment only after the condition has become aggravated. Minor imbalances cannot be detected using such methods. In the case of yoga practitioners, a self-awareness of one's body and its imbalances are heightened through daily yoga practice; as a result, minor imbalances can be identified and addressed.

Once you have established a firm and balanced foundation in your asana practice, you will be able to progress to the next step—the balance of breath and mind.

In Chapter 1, we will look at the various methods you can use to intuitively identify imbalances through yoga poses.

All Imbalances Have an Order

Before we can correct an imbalance, we need to understand its cause. If we cannot see the repeated pattern in the yoga poses, we cannot identify what must be corrected. Fortunately, there is an order, even in complex imbalances, seen in yoga postures.

Basic Yoga Patterns: Forward and Backward Bends

The basic yoga poses are made up of forward and backward bending positions. These poses are important, as they enable the practitioner to be aware of his/her own imbalances in either the front or the back line of the body.

Forward bends lengthen the back of the body, while backward bends lengthen the front. One does not need extensive training to feel these sensations. We often feel some level of muscle ache when we stretch.

Figure 1.1 shows various forward bending yoga poses with different foundations: standing, sitting, and lying (inverted) on the ground.

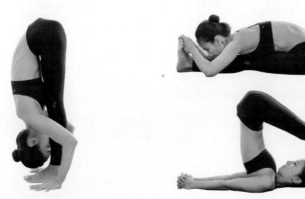

Figure 1.1. *Forward bending yoga poses.*

Backward bending yoga poses require the body to bend backward, pushing it outward and upward, lengthening areas such as the chest, stomach, pelvis, and thighs.

Figure 1.2 demonstrates various backward bending yoga poses with different directions and foundations: lying, sitting, and inverted.

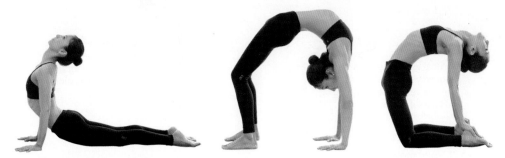

Figure 1.2. *Backward bending yoga poses.*

Basic Joint Movement Patterns: Flexion and Extension

If you study the above yoga poses, you may notice that they have been created around movements of the joints. There is a standard pattern in the joints' movements as the human body moves in a particular direction or enters a pose.

In forward bending positions, the cervical, thoracic, and lumbar vertebrae, as well as the hip joints, are flexed in a forward direction (in the sagittal plane). Conversely, in backward bending positions, the hip joints and the lumbar, thoracic, and cervical vertebrae are extended in a backward direction (in the sagittal plane).

In other words, the forward bend poses form part of the flexion patterns, while the backward bend poses are part of the extension patterns.

Flexion and Extension Movements of the Joints

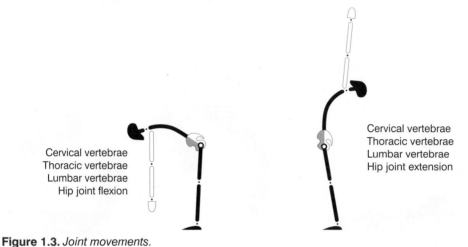

Cervical vertebrae
Thoracic vertebrae
Lumbar vertebrae
Hip joint flexion

Cervical vertebrae
Thoracic vertebrae
Lumbar vertebrae
Hip joint extension

Figure 1.3. *Joint movements.*

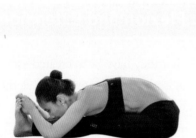

Figure 1.4. *Forward bending pose: flexion pattern.*

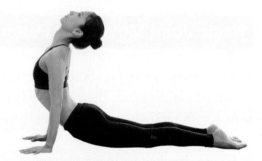

Figure 1.5. *Backward bending pose: extension pattern.*

Patterns of Balanced and Unbalanced Poses

If you observed the flexion and extension of the cervical, thoracic, and lumbar vertebrae during the movements of the joints, you will be able to identify the imbalances in the forward and backward bending poses.

When the various joints of the cervical, thoracic, or lumbar spine and the hips are evenly flexed in a forward bend pose, we would view this as a balanced forward bend.

However, when some of the joints are over-flexed while others are insufficiently flexed, most of the weight and effort will be carried out by these few specific over-flexed joints. This will result in an imbalance.

Through the synergized movement of muscles and joints, the front and back joints can flex and extend evenly, creating balanced forward or backward bending poses. When only a specific set of joints is frequently being used, however, imbalances will arise because of the lack of use of the other joints.

Unfortunately, not only in daily activities but also during yoga practice, practitioners often maintain their bad habits of unbalanced forward and backward bend poses. **As there are relatively more forward and backward bending postures in yoga than any other directional poses, continued practice with imbalances in specific joints will usually compound these imbalances.**

Where our movements become habitual, any imbalance may go unnoticed, as we perform these movements unconsciously. In addition, the body keeps on favoring the use of one set of joints and neglecting another, leading to their weakening.

Line and Section Imbalances

The actual movements of the body are rather different from those illustrated in anatomy books. A single muscle does not operate in isolation, but as a part of the synchronous action of a combination of muscle structures, interconnected with the fasciae.

When a person bends forward, the hamstrings are not the only muscles to be lengthened. Every part of the back side of the body is affected—starting from the forehead and continuing through the cervical, thoracic, and lumbar spines, the gluteus, and the hamstrings, to the soles of the feet. The whole extended back side of the body will form, in this case, the back line. In contrast, when the body is bending backward, the front muscles, which are being stretched, will form the contiguous front line.

Obviously, there are many more links between the joints and the muscles of the body, including the lateral and spiral lines of the body (for a detailed analysis, see *Anatomy Trains* by Tom Myers*). But, if we understand the connection between the two main lines (the back and front lines), we can identify the cause of the imbalances of the front and back sides of the body. (I am also in the process of writing a book on the symmetric imbalance of the lateral and spiral lines.)

Figure 1.6 depicts four important sections of joints along the back and front lines of the body.

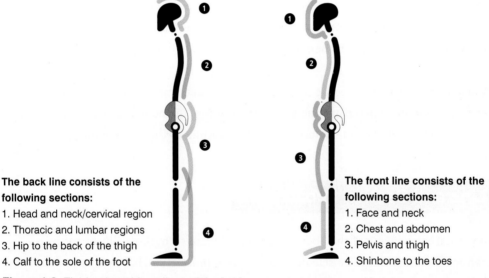

The back line consists of the following sections:
1. Head and neck/cervical region
2. Thoracic and lumbar regions
3. Hip to the back of the thigh
4. Calf to the sole of the foot

The front line consists of the following sections:
1. Face and neck
2. Chest and abdomen
3. Pelvis and thigh
4. Shinbone to the toes

Figure 1.6. *The back and front lines of the body.*

Why did we divide the front and back line into the simple four sections rather than into joints and muscles? Simply because these four sections are already divided by the major joints of the body, representing a practical functional unit.

The human body is made up of 206 bones, over 400 skeletal muscles, and more than 230 movable and semi-movable joints. When we observe yoga poses during their

*Myers, T.W. 2014. *Anatomy Trains*, Churchill Livingstone: Edinburgh.

practice, we realize that the conventional tools, such as X-ray or muscle testing, for examining postural imbalances are not practical. Accordingly, we look for simple tools to use on our yoga mats.

For doctors and therapists, those conventional methods are essential. The patient can totally passively relax while the physical therapist palpates each joint and muscle separately. During yoga practice, however, no single muscle or joint acts in isolation; in fact, several muscles and joints work together like a single functional unit. That is why dividing the sections, which are made up of the major joints like the hip and spine, is practical. We can move cervical joints without moving thoracic and lumbar joints; however, when we move for example the thoracic or lumbar joints, we must move some of the other joints as well. This is the reason why we can divide the whole spine into two sections, where the cervical region is a separate functional unit, and the thoracic and lumbar regions together form another functional unit.

Section 1 has at least 8 movable joints, but when we move, all cervical joints work as one functional unit to perform flexion or extension.

Section 2 has at least 17 joints, but when we move, all thoracic and lumbar joints again work as one functional unit to flex or extend the spine.

Section 3 comprises the hip joint and sacroiliac joint; the latter is semi-movable and should therefore not move, in order to provide stability to the pelvis.

Section 4 has at least 16 movable joints, but the ankle joint is the most important one to ensure dorsiflexion and plantar flexion of the foot.

The knee joint is located between Sections 3 and 4.

If the forward bending poses are easier to perform than the backward bending poses, the back line is relatively effectively lengthened, as demonstrated in Figure 1.7, while the front line is less so, representing an imbalance, as illustrated in Figure 1.8.

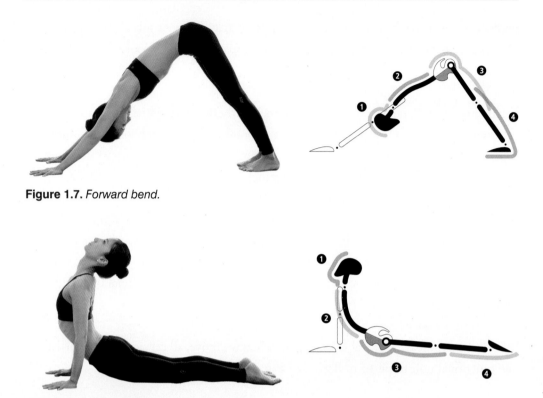

Figure 1.7. *Forward bend.*

Figure 1.8. *Backward bend.*

In general, if the forward bend postures are easier to perform than the backward bend postures, we can safely assume that the back line is better lengthened than the front line. This may indicate a line imbalance.

In other words, imbalances can manifest through the whole structure of the front or back side of the body. In many such cases, a safe generic solution to correct a line imbalance would be to practice more of either forward or backward bending poses, whichever are more challenging.

Sections are parts of the front and back lines as defined above. A section imbalance is even more common than a line imbalance. In a section imbalance, there is a significant difference in the ability to lengthen the muscles of a specific section compared with the muscles in the other sections of the same line. When we learn to observe sectional imbalances, we can identify certain sets of joints and muscle imbalances, which represent one of the main causes of postural imbalances.

Single-section vs. Multi-section Poses

By and large, if you compare various yoga poses, single-section poses lengthen only one section of the line and are relatively easier than multi-section poses, which lengthen more than one section.

Let us take a single-section pose—the Cow or Cat pose, shown in Figures 1.9 and 1.10. This asana requires the knees to be bent, lengthening only Section 2 of the back line (thoracic and lumbar regions). It is comfortable, even for beginners.

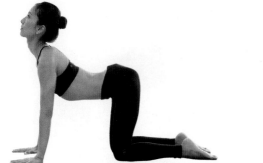 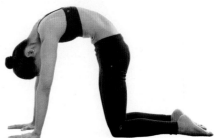

Figure 1.9. *Cow pose (Bitilasana).*   **Figure 1.10.** *Cat pose (Marjaryasana).*

A multi-section pose, such as a Downward-facing dog (Figure 1.11), requires the knees to be straight, which can result in tension in several sections: Section 2 (thoracic and lumbar regions), Section 3 (gluteal muscles and back of the upper leg), and Section 4 (the calf and the bottom of the feet).

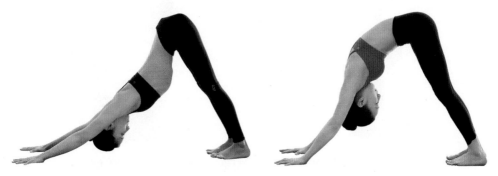

Figure 1.11. *Imbalances in Downward-facing dog pose (Adho Mukha Svanasana).*

It is very common to see practitioners with a shortened Section 2 (Figure 1.11, left image) of the back line, or Section 3 (Figure 1.11, right image) of the back line. Such fixed, unbalanced conditions of these sections challenge free movement of the lumbar and pelvic areas.

Looking into the other single-section poses, for example Hero (Figure 1.12) and Bound angle (Figure 1.13) poses, we see that the fully bent knees result in easy lengthening of a single section—extension and flexion of Section 2 (thoracic and lumbar regions).

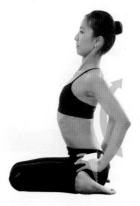 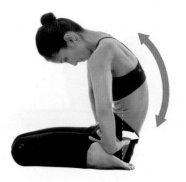

Figure 1.12. *Hero pose (Virasana).*

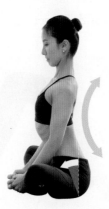 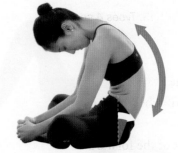

Figure 1.13. *Bound angle pose (Baddha Konasana B).*

For the sake of this investigation, we can also transform the seated single-section pose into a multi-section pose by extending the knees. When the tension exerted on the body is increased, the spine will curve into a C or D shape depending on the postural type (A or P).

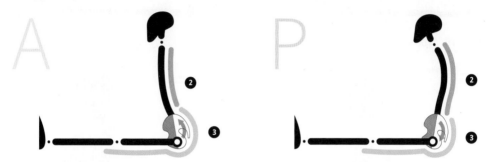

Figure 1.14. *Left: Type A—short Section 2 and long Section 3. Right: Type P—long Section 2 and short Section 3.*

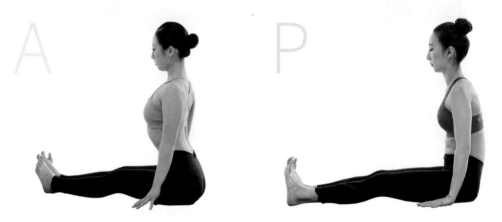

Figure 1.15. *Types A and P in Staff pose (Dandasana).*

In the multi-section pose depicted in Figures 1.16 and 1.17, you might be able to identify the unbalanced joints by comparing the relative lengths of Sections 2 and 3.

Most of the forward and backward bending yoga poses are multi-section poses, which extend to more than just a single section of the body.

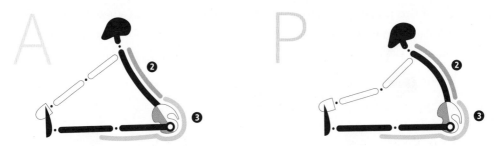

Figure 1.16. *Types A and P in Seated forward bend.*

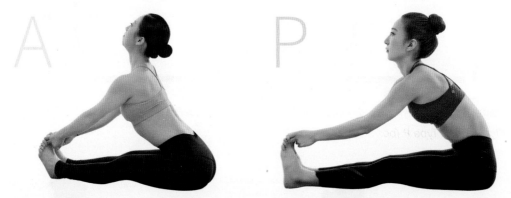

Figure 1.17. *Types A and P in Seated forward bend/Western stretch (Paschimottanasana).*

Observation of Multi-section Forward Bend Poses

Seated Forward Bend Pose (Paschimottanasana)

Figure 1.18 shows an unbalanced Seated forward bend pose which mainly lengthens the back line of Section 3, while Figure 1.19 shows an unbalanced pose which mainly lengthens the back line of Section 2. Figure 1.20, on the other hand, demonstrates the lengthening of both Sections 2 and 3 of the back line, which is an example of a balanced forward bend.

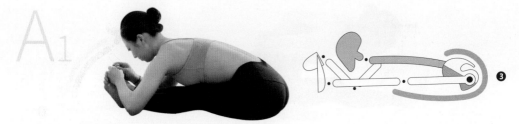

Figure 1.18. *Type A (anterior pelvic tilt).*

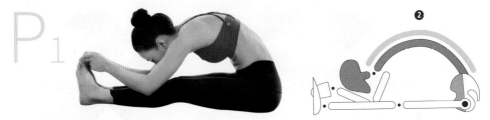

Figure 1.19. *Type P (posterior pelvic tilt).*

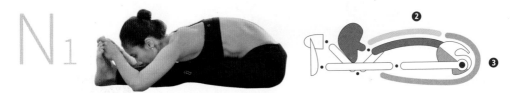

Figure 1.20. *Type N (neutral pelvic tilt).*

Sage Marichi Pose A (Marichyasana A)

Figure 1.21 shows an unbalanced Sage Marichi pose A which lengthens mainly Section 3, while Figure 1.22 shows the unbalanced pose in which mainly only Section 2 is lengthened. Figure 1.23 demonstrates a balanced Sage Marichi pose A, with Sections 2 and 3 being lengthened simultaneously.

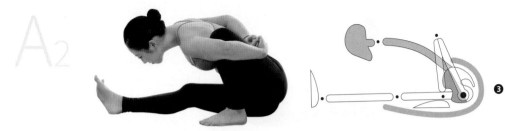

Figure 1.21. *Type A (anterior pelvic tilt).*

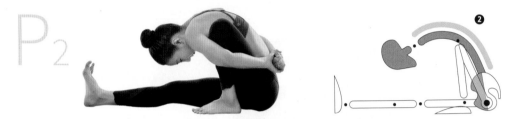

Figure 1.22. *Type P (posterior pelvic tilt).*

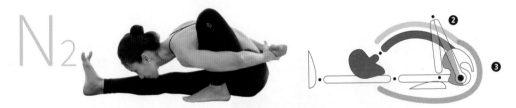

Figure 1.23. *Type N (neutral pelvic tilt).*

Tortoise Pose (Kurmasana)

Figure 1.24 shows an unbalanced Tortoise pose which only lengthens Section 3. The lumbar region of Section 2 looks almost straight, as if it is not being lengthened at all. Additionally, the foundation of the sit bones is weakened, as a result of the extreme lengthening of Section 3, and the practitioner is unable to raise their feet off the ground.

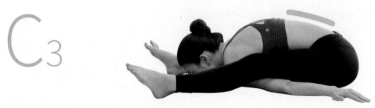

Figure 1.24. *Type C (complex).*

On the other hand, the curve around the lumbar area of Section 2 in Figure 1.25 shows the lengthening of both Sections 2 and 3 of the back line. Here, Type N illustrates a balanced Tortoise pose, whereby the sit bones are allowed to stay close to the ground, hence facilitating the strength to be able to pick the feet up off the ground.

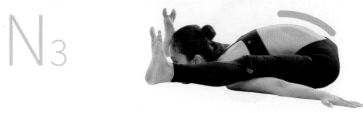

Figure 1.25. *Type N (neutral).*

From the above examples, we can see that with multi-section forward bending postures, if only a single section is lengthened, the probability of this particular section becoming overstretched and the other section becoming stiffened is high. This situation will eventually lead to pain, and the risk of sustaining an injury will increase.

In order to progress to the next level of multi-section poses such as the Tortoise pose and the Sleeping tortoise pose, the lengthening of both Sections 2 and 3 simultaneously by means of the simpler forward bend poses is an absolute prerequisite.

Sleeping Tortoise Pose (Supta Kurmasana)

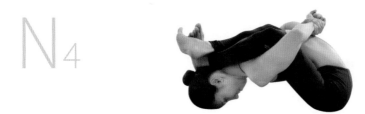

Figure 1.26. *Type N (neutral).*

When Sections 2 and 3 are lengthened together, the foundation of the sit bones can be established, bringing about a balance to the Sleeping tortoise pose (Figure 1.26).

Two Feet Behind the Head Pose (Dvi Pada Sirsasana)

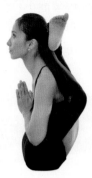

Figure 1.27. *Type N (neutral).*

When the spine is curved sufficiently, the lengthening of Section 2 is evident. Both Sections 2 and 3 are balancing and lengthening. Counteraction of the crossed legs and the spine, while keeping the sit bones firmly planted on the ground, ensures a high level of balance in the Two feet behind the head pose (Figure 1.27).

Observation of Multi-section Backward Bending Poses

Upward-facing Dog Pose (Urdhva Mukha Svanasana)

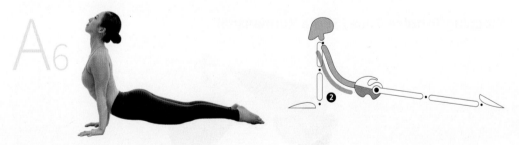

Figure 1.28. *Type A (anterior).*

Figure 1.28 shows an unbalanced Upward-facing dog pose which mainly lengthens Section 2 (chest and abdomen) of the front line. Section 3 (pelvis, front of upper leg) is insufficiently lengthened. From the lifted tailbone and the big gap between the hips and the ground, we can postulate that the posterior pelvic tilt has not been developed properly; this leads to the insufficient lengthening of Section 3 of the front line.

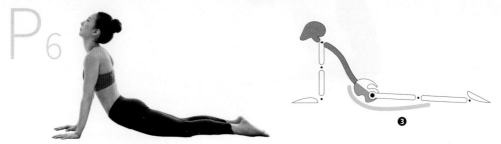

Figure 1.29. *Type P (posterior).*

Figure 1.29 shows an unbalanced Upward-facing dog pose which mainly lengthens Section 3 (pelvis, front of upper leg) of the front line, but not Section 2. Contrary to Figure 1.28, here the tucked-in tailbone and a small gap between the hips and the ground tells us that the posterior pelvic tilt is achieved; however, the insufficient curvature of the lumbar region leads to the limited lengthening of the front line of Section 2.

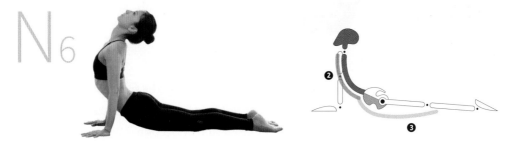

Figure 1.30. *Type N (neutral).*

Figure 1.30 shows both Sections 2 and 3 of the front line lengthening together in a well-balanced backward bend.

Camel Pose (Ustrasana)

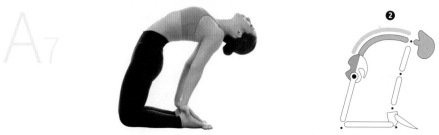

Figure 1.31. *Type A.*

Figure 1.31 shows an unbalanced Camel pose where Section 2 of the front line is lengthening well, whereas Section 3 is not. In addition, the tailbone remains lifted, restricting sufficient forward movement of the pelvis, which would have created a stronger foundation of the feet.

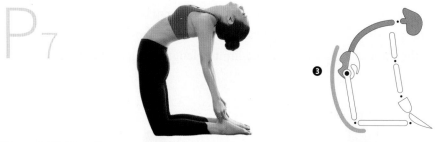

Figure 1.32. *Type P.*

Figure 1.32 shows an unbalanced Camel pose where mainly the front line of Section 3 (pelvis, front of upper leg) is lengthened but not Section 2. Contrary to Figure 1.31, the tailbone is tucked in sufficiently, and the front line of Section 3 (pelvis, front of upper leg) is efficiently lengthened. The front line of Section 2 (chest and abdomen), however, is not adequately expanded and lengthened.

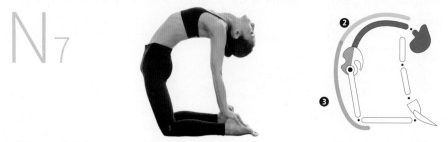

Figure 1.33. *Type N.*

Figure 1.33 shows both Sections 2 and 3 of the front of the body lengthening together in a well-balanced backward bend pose.

Upward Bow Pose (Urdhva Dhanurasana)

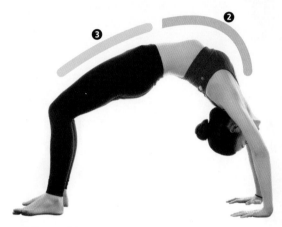

Figure 1.34. *Unbalanced Upward bow pose.*

Figure 1.34 demonstrates an unbalanced multi-section Upward bow pose where Section 2 of the front line is relatively well lengthened, whereas Section 3 is not.

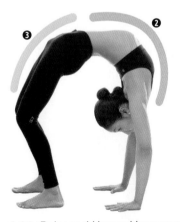
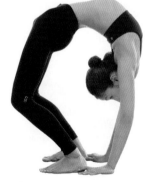

Figure 1.35. *Balanced Upward bow pose.*

Figure 1.35 shows the collaborative extension of the lumbar region and the hip joints. This allows Sections 2 and 3 of the front line to lengthen evenly and enter a deep and well-balanced backward bend without pain or risk of injury.

Drop Back Preparation Pose

Figure 1.36 shows the lumbar extension. Figure 1.37 shows the excessive hip joint extension in an unbalanced backward bending pose.

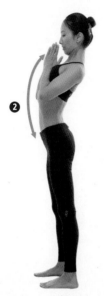

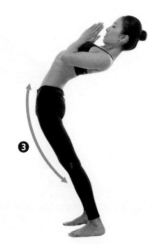

Figure 1.36. *Extension of the lumbar joints, lengthening Section 2 of the front line.*

Figure 1.37. *Extension of the hip joint, lengthening Section 3 of the front line.*

Figure 1.38 demonstrates the balanced backward bend preparation pose (Drop back pose), with the lumbar region and hip joint extending simultaneously.

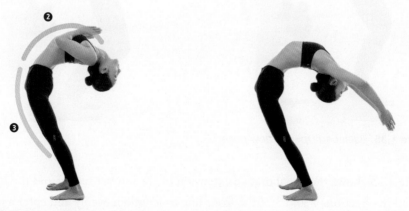

Figure 1.38. *Balanced Drop back preparation pose, with Sections 2 and 3 of the front line lengthening together.*

Scorpion Pose (Vrschikasana) and Lord of the Dance Pose (Natarajasana)

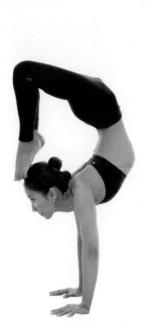

Figure 1.39. *Scorpion pose (Vrschikasana).*

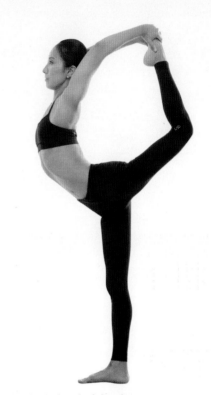

Figure 1.40. *Lord of the dance pose (Natarajasana).*

Figures 1.39 and 1.40 also demonstrate the lumbar and hip joints extending together in balanced backward bending poses—Scorpion and Lord of the dance.

Both Sections 2 and 3 are lengthening simultaneously, representing stable, balanced multi-section backward bending poses.

2

Understanding Spinal and Lumbopelvic Anatomy

So far, we have explored forward and backward bending yoga asanas and the methods for identifying imbalances in the front and back lines of the body. We have also looked at the imbalances in sections of the body. Through observing asanas and comparing specific imbalances along the sections of the body, we can easily identify imbalances in the spine and pelvic areas. I hope that you will find this technique intuitive and useful.

The observational method of the yoga asana practitioner is akin to looking at a forest. By combining the technique of observing the "forest" of a human body intuitively with the method of observing a "tree" anatomically in terms of the bones, joints, and muscles, a more systematic analysis of the imbalances can be achieved.

When we look at structural imbalances, an understanding of the musculoskeletal system and its functions is essential for the accurate reading of the imbalances in joint movement.

This chapter contains some level of anatomical detail, but I have tried to present it as simply as possible. Learning a bit more about muscle imbalances, while understanding the shape and causes of an unbalanced spine and pelvis, will help you to make deeper and more precise analyses.

Key Points in Observing the Spine: Curvature and Primary and Secondary Curves

Anatomy books and classes frequently teach us that an S-shaped curvature of the spine is important. Abnormalities, such as lordosis of the lumbar spine or kyphosis of the thoracic spine, are excessive curvatures of the spine.

The shape of a normal, upright adult spine is a natural S-shaped curve, made up of 26 spinal joints. A normal cervical spine, consisting of seven vertebrae, forms a concave C-shaped curve at the top of the back. On the upper back of the body, a normal twelve-joint thoracic spine forms a convex D curve. This is followed by the five-joint lumbar spine, which forms a natural concave C curve. Below the lumbar spine are the sacrum and coccyx, which make up the final convex D-shaped curve at the base of the spine.

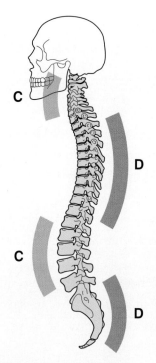

Figure 2.1. *Adult spine.*

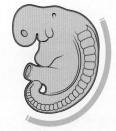

Figure 2.2. *Embryo/fetus spine.*

The C-shaped curves in the cervical and lumbar regions are known as *lordotic* or *secondary curves*, while the D-shaped curves in the thoracic and sacral regions are known as *kyphotic* or *primary curves*.

The reason why the D-shaped curves are referred to as *primary* curves and the C-shaped curves are referred to as *secondary* curves lies in the anatomy of the embryo/ fetus development. An embryo's spine is first formed in the mother's womb and is curved like the letter D. The secondary curves in the cervical and lumbar regions are developed only after birth.

A yoga asana that depicts these primary curves is Pindasana (Embryo or Fetus pose). Cow pose focuses on the secondary curves.

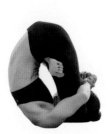

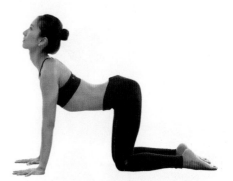

Figure 2.3. *Fetus pose (Pindasana). Emphasis is on primary curves.*

Figure 2.4. *Cow pose (Bitilasana). Emphasis is on secondary curves.*

Depending on the asana, our natural curve shapes may shift so that D-shaped curves (primary curves) become C-shaped curves (secondary curves), and vice versa. In addition, a practitioner's postural type may result in shifts in the curves.

Figure 2.5 demonstrates clear extension of the lumbar spine (Type A), while Figure 2.6 demonstrates flexion of the lumbar spine (Type P).

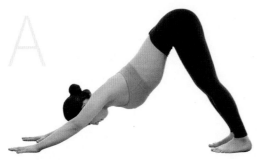

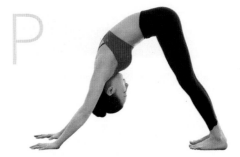

Figure 2.5. *Type A: Downward-facing dog pose (Adho Mukha Svanasana).*

Figure 2.6. *Type P: Downward-facing dog pose (Adho Mukha Svanasana).*

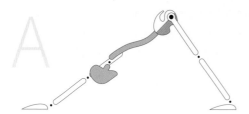

Figure 2.7. *Type A: Downward-facing dog pose.*

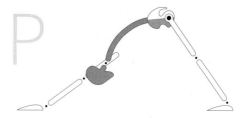

Figure 2.8. *Type P: Downward-facing dog pose.*

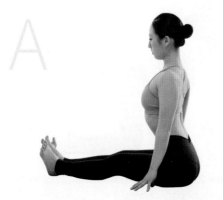

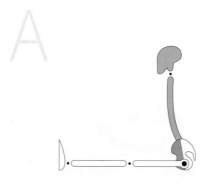

Figure 2.9. *Type A: Staff pose (Dandasana).*

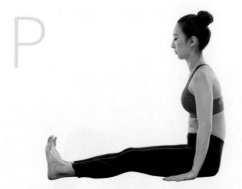

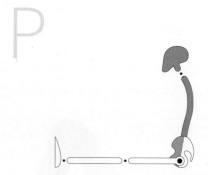

Figure 2.10. *Type P: Staff pose (Dandasana).*

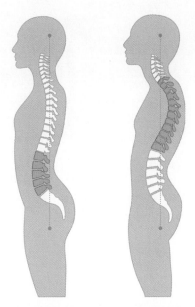

Figure 2.11. *Lordosis and kyphosis of the spine.*

Understanding the Relationship Between the Spinal Curves and Pelvic Tilt

Most cases of an unbalanced spinal curvature are linked to an unbalanced pelvic tilt. Imagine the spine as a column and the pelvis as a plinth; if the pelvis starts tilting, the spine will also change its position.

Type A in Figure 2.12 demonstrates lordosis (excessive inward curvature of the lumbar spine). It is fairly common for people with lordosis to develop an exaggerated anterior pelvic tilt.

In contrast, Type P in Figure 2.12 demonstrates kyphosis (excessive outward curvature of the thoracic spine). People with this condition often suffer from a significant posterior pelvic tilt.

The orientation of the pelvic tilt can be determined by looking at the horizontal alignment of the yoga pants in Figure 2.13.

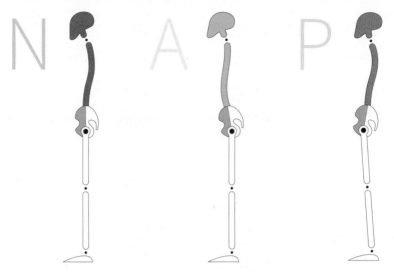

Figure 2.12. *Spinal curvatures: N, A, P—neutral, lordosis, kyphosis.*

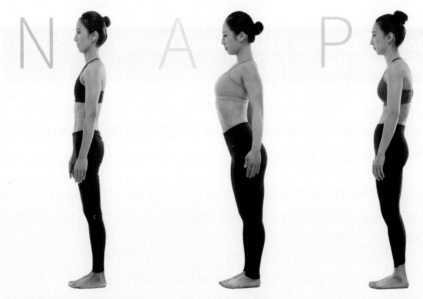

Figure 2.13. *Pelvic tilt: N, A, P (normal, lordosis, kyphosis).*

In anatomical terms, the pelvis is in a neutral position when the anterior superior iliac spine (ASIS), a small bony projection at the upper front of the ilium, is in vertical alignment with the pubic crest.

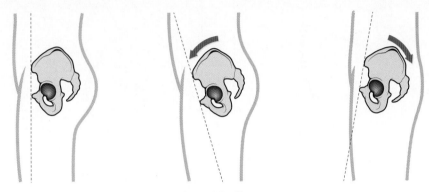

Figure 2.14. *Neutral, anterior, and posterior pelvic tilts.*

Q1 What Is the Difference Between Hip Flexion/ Extension and Pelvic Tilt, and What Are the Unbalanced States of Pelvic Tilt?

Hip Flexion and Anterior Pelvic Tilt

The plane that divides the body into left and right portions is called the *sagittal plane*. *Hip flexion* refers to the movement of the **femur** relative to the pelvis, while *anterior pelvic tilt* refers to the movement of the **pelvis** relative to the femur **within the sagittal plane.**

Both hip flexion and anterior pelvic tilt occur at the hip joint, reducing the angle of this joint, brought about by the muscle contraction of the hip flexors, e.g., the psoas. However, there is a difference between those two movements. *Hip flexion* is the anterior movement of the femur as the insertion of the psoas moves toward the lumbar region and pelvis at the origins of the psoas. *Anterior pelvic tilt* is the movement of the lumbar region and pelvis, where the origin of the psoas moves toward the femur at its own insertion.

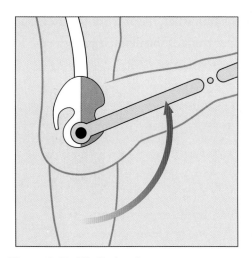

Figure 2.15. *Hip flexion (femur movement).*

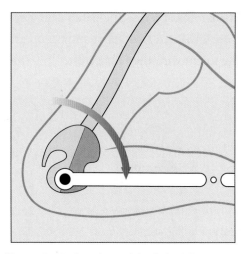

Figure 2.16. *Anterior pelvic tilt (pelvis movement).*

Usually, beginners are more at ease with hip flexion than with anterior pelvic tilt movement, because of a myriad of reasons, such as physical habits, instincts, and activities they have been engaging in from childhood. Through practicing a new direction of movement with the same muscle group, anterior pelvic tilt can be improved. In yoga, therefore, we usually talk about **awakening the psoas**, rather than strengthening it for those who already have a strong psoas muscle.

Hip Extension and Posterior Pelvic Tilt

Hip extension, which takes place in the sagittal plane, is the movement of the femur, while posterior pelvic tilt is the movement of the pelvis.

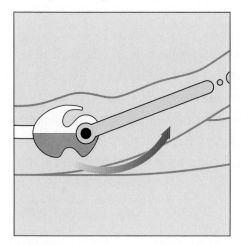

Figure 2.17. *Hip extension (femur movement).*

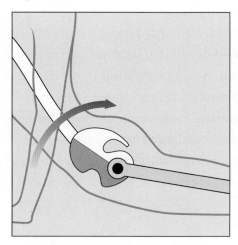

Figure 2.18. *Posterior pelvic tilt (pelvis movement).*

Hip extension and *posterior pelvic tilt* refer to the movements of the hip joint using the same muscles but in different directions; in other words, the main hip extensor, the gluteus maximus, acts in both hip extension and posterior pelvic tilt.

The movement of the femur (and the insertion of the gluteus maximus) toward the pelvis (and the origin of the gluteal muscles), however, is known as *hip extension*. On the other hand, the movement of the pelvis (and origin of the gluteus maximus) toward the insertion or iliotibial tract on the femur, is known as *posterior pelvic tilt*.

In summary, anterior pelvic tilt is considered a hip flexion, because the essence of its motion is the same, even though its subject (the pelvis) is different from that of the original hip flexion (the femur). Therefore, it is common to have both hip flexion and anterior pelvic tilt in a flexion movement of the hip joint.

Posterior pelvic tilt is considered a hip extension, as the essence of its joint motion is the same, even though its subject (the pelvis) is different from that of the original hip extension (the femur). Basically, there is both hip extension and posterior pelvic tilt in an extension movement of the hip joint.

Pelvic Tilt and Pelvic Tilt Imbalances

As mentioned above, both anterior pelvic tilt and posterior pelvic tilt are movements of the joints which are commonly required in yoga asanas. During our daily lives or in many sports, it is common for the pelvis to be in a fixed position and for the femur to move into hip flexion or extension. In contrast, in yoga asanas, it is also common for the femur to be in fixed position and for the pelvis to tilt anteriorly or posteriorly. The muscles used for these actions are the same, but their direction of execution is different. The major reason for such yoga movements is to correct imbalances in anterior and posterior pelvic tilt. For example, for those with an anteriorly unbalanced pelvis, it is advised to practice a posterior pelvic tilt rather than working from the hip and moving the femur. Yoga asanas simply teach us to work with the pelvis directly rather than with the femur, if we have pelvic imbalances.

For those with a neutral pelvis, an anterior or posterior pelvic tilt is normal movement during a sitting or standing position. For those with a non-neutral pelvis, however, a pelvic tilt presents an imbalance; as a consequence, anterior and posterior tilt imbalances would already exist in both flexion and extension of the hip joint, and are likely to result in overall spine, and ultimately postural, imbalances.

Anterior pelvic tilt imbalance = an unbalanced state in hip flexion.

Posterior pelvic tilt imbalance = an unbalanced state in hip extension.

The causes of the imbalances of the lumbar curvature and pelvic tilt are often found in the imbalances of the core muscles.

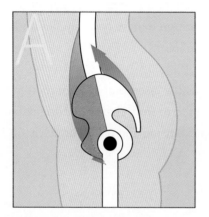

Figure 2.19. *Type A: Anterior pelvic tilt = hip flexion + lumbar extension. Psoas and erector spinae muscles are locked-short and strong.*

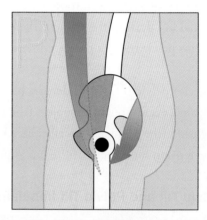

Figure 2.20. *Type P: Posterior pelvic tilt = hip extension + lumbar flexion. Rectus abdominis and gluteus maximus muscles are locked-short and strong.*

Four Core Muscles That Control Lumbopelvic Balance

An imbalance of the core muscles, caused by long-term postural habits, is both a cause and an effect of the spine and pelvic tilt pattern.

Let us look in detail at Type A, with shortened and stiffened psoas and erector spinae, followed by Type P, with shortened rectus abdominis and gluteus maximus.

Type A is a condition where the psoas (which is the deep core muscle used in hip flexion) and the erector spinae (which extend the lumbar region) are stiffened and shortened (locked-short). As a result, an unbalanced postural alignment appears as anterior pelvic tilt (hip flexion) and excessive lumbar extension (lordosis).

Type P is a condition where the rectus abdominis (which flexes the lumbar region) and the gluteus maximus (which extends the hip joints) become shortened and stiffened (locked-short). As a result, an unbalanced postural alignment appears as posterior pelvic tilt (hip extension) and lumbar flexion.

Four core muscles are depicted in Figure 2.21. The psoas and rectus abdominis muscles are located in front of the body, and the gluteus maximus and erector spinae are at the back of the body.

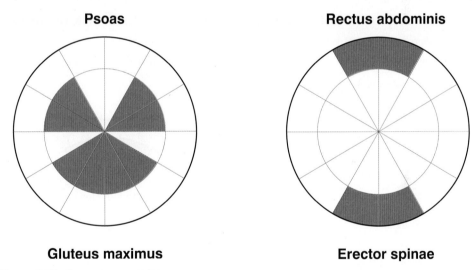

Figure 2.21. *Four core muscles.*

The inner circle in Figure 2.21, made up of core muscles such as the psoas and gluteus maximus muscles, represents deep muscles. The outer circle, made up of the rectus abdominis muscles and erector spinae, depicts superficial muscles.

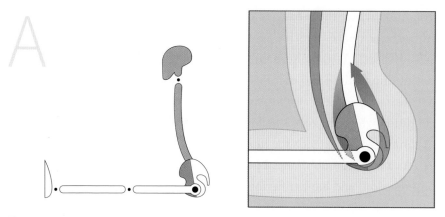

Figure 2.22. *Type A anterior pelvic tilt and the core muscles. Locked-short (blue): psoas, erector spinae. Locked-long (red): gluteus maximus, rectus abdominis.*

In Type A, since the pelvis is already leaning forward when standing or sitting, the hip flexors—such as the psoas and rectus femoris—are shortened. In addition, the lumbar extensor erector spinae muscles are also shortened (locked-short or hypertonic). On the other hand, the hip extensors—such as the gluteus maximus, hamstrings, and rectus abdominis—are lengthened (locked-long).

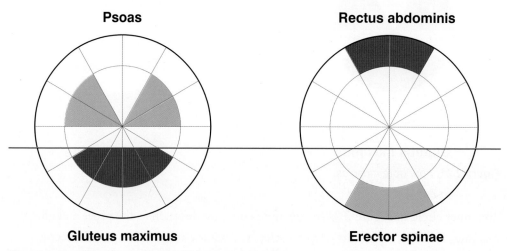

Figure 2.23. *Effect of anterior tilt on the core muscles.*

The red horizontal line in Figure 2.23 shows the effect of anterior pelvic tilt on the core muscles. The gluteus maximus is not functioning properly as a hip extensor and is weakened, which results in an imbalance in anterior tilt.

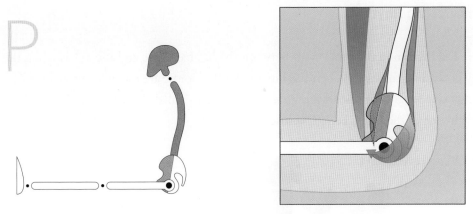

Figure 2.24. *Type P posterior pelvic tilt and the core muscles. Locked-short (blue): rectus abdominis, gluteus maximus. Locked-long (red): psoas, erector spinae.*

In contrast, for Type P, as the pelvis is already tilting backward in a standing position, the hip extensors, such as the gluteus maximus and hamstrings, are shortened (locked-short). Not only that, the rectus abdominis—the lumbar spine flexor—is also shortened. In addition, the hip flexors, such as the psoas, rectus femoris, and erector spinae, are lengthened and locked in that condition.

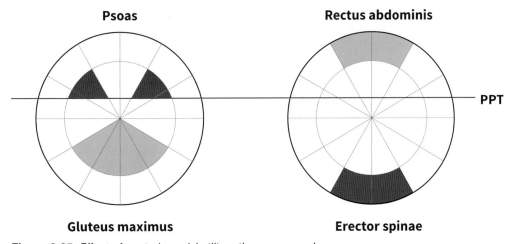

Figure 2.25. *Effect of posterior pelvic tilt on the core muscles.*

The red horizontal line in Figure 2.25 shows the effect of posterior pelvic tilt on the core muscles. The psoas is not functioning properly and is weak, which results in a posterior tilt imbalance.

Lumbopelvic Rhythm

There is a rhythm in the movement between the lumbar spine and the pelvis when the body is bending forward. When the hip and lumbar joints are moving in synchronicity, a well-balanced forward bend can be achieved, but an unbalanced forward bend will result in one of the joints being overused.

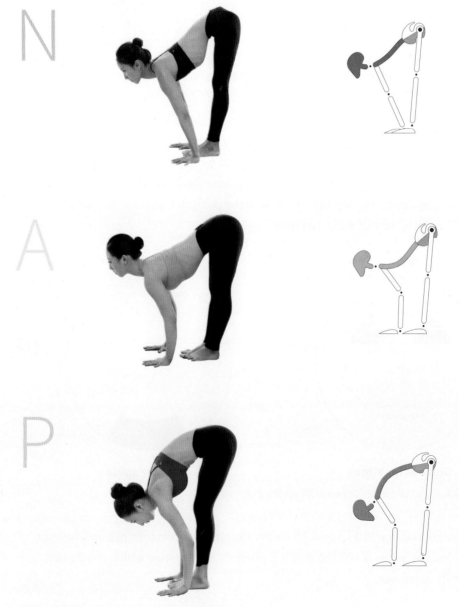

Figure 2.26. *Lumbopelvic rhythm patterns.*

If just either the lumbar joints or the hip joints are used in the movement, the unbalanced condition may worsen instead of improving.

The hip and lumbar joints work together in forward and backward bends. However, if a certain muscle is shortened and stiffened (locked-short) and only the hip joint or the lumbar joint is used, the passive joint will weaken.

In Type A, the forward lumbar curve is excessive and there is a severe unbalanced pattern of anterior pelvic tilt. Type A uses mainly the hip joint, since the psoas and erector spinae muscles are shortened.

The hip flexor of the short and strong psoas is habitually used first in the Standing half forward bend preparation pose (Ardha Uttanasana—Figure 2.27) or in the Seated forward bend pose (Paschimottanasana—Figure 2.28).

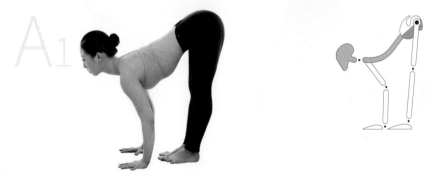

Figure 2.27. *Type A: Standing half forward bend preparation pose (Ardha Uttanasana).*

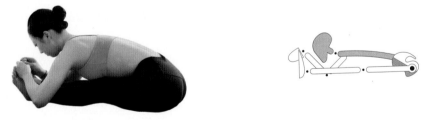

Figure 2.28. *Type A: Seated forward bend pose (Paschimottanasana).*

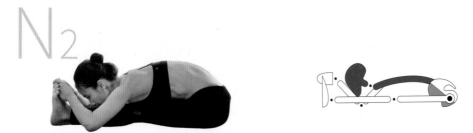

Figure 2.29. *Type N: Seated forward bend pose (Paschimottanasana).*

The original intention of a Seated forward bend is a flexion of not only the hip joint but also the lumbar region, as it is lengthening the entire back line from the sole of the foot to the forehead (Figure 2.29). If, habitually, only hip flexion occurs, as in Type A, the pattern of imbalance may worsen.

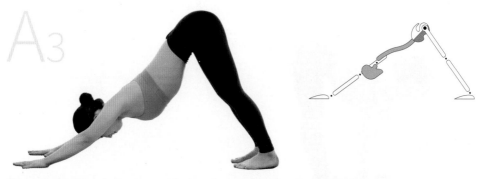

Figure 2.30. *Type A: Downward-facing dog pose (Adho Mukha Svanasana).*

In Downward-facing dog (Adho Mukha Svanasana) there is no likelihood of lengthening the lumbar region by flexion, as usually only lumbar extension and hip flexion will occur (Figure 2.30).

For Type A, the main driver in backward bends is lumbar extension, since these extensors are strong and shortened. It is also difficult to perform hip extension because of the resistance from the strong and short hip flexor (psoas) and relatively weak hip extensors (gluteus maximus, hamstrings).

For example, when Type A attempts the Upward-facing dog pose (Figure 2.31) or the Camel pose (Figure 2.32), the lumbar region naturally takes most of the load. Due to the unbalanced muscles and habits, the pubic bone automatically moves down while the tailbone moves up, leading to an anterior pelvic tilt imbalance. Ultimately, hip extension is interrupted, as hip flexion occurs first and takes over.

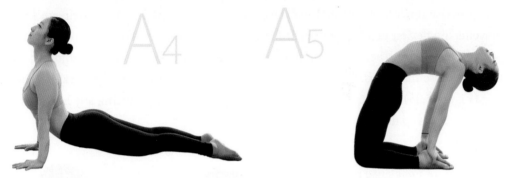

Figure 2.31. *Type A: Upward-facing dog pose (Urdhva Mukha Svanasana).*   **Figure 2.32.** *Type A: Camel pose (Ustrasana).*

The lumbar and hip joints are required to work together to execute a balanced backward bend. In Type A, however, only lumbar extension is active, leaving the extension of the hip joint inactive. If, through habit, only the lumbar area is used during a backward bend, the erector spinae will become stiffened and shortened. As a result, anterior pelvic tilt (APT) will become more profound, resulting in back pain.

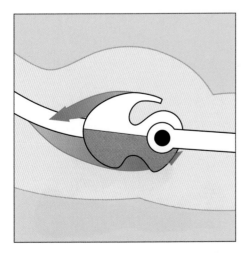 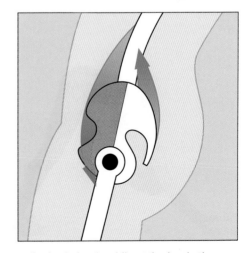

Figure 2.33. *At the front, the psoas is short and strong (locked-short), while at the back, the erector spinae are short and strong (locked-short).*

On the other hand, an unbalanced pattern based only on lumbar flexion is likely to happen in forward bend asanas with Type P.

Type P has difficulty in adequately flexing the hip joint, because of inactive hip flexors (the psoas) and relatively strong hip extensors (gluteus maximus and hamstrings). This prevents hip flexion in a Standing half forward bend (Figure 2.34) or a Seated forward bend (Figure 2.36). There is a rounding of the spine, which flexes the lumbar joints; this is because the rectus abdominis is relatively short and strong. In Downward-facing dog (Figure 2.35), lumbar flexion will usually be initiated first, reducing any likelihood of satisfactory hip flexion.

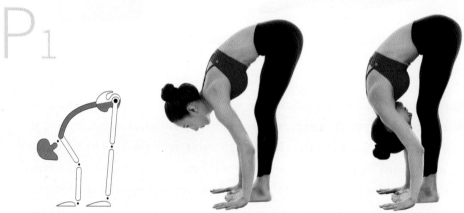

Figure 2.34. *Type P: Standing half forward bend preparation pose (Ardha Uttanasana).*

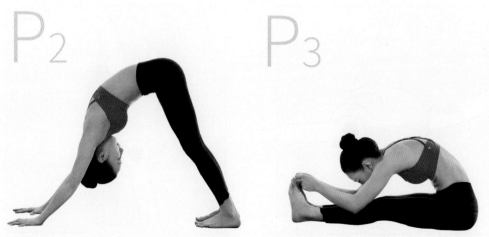

Figure 2.35. *Type P: Downward-facing dog pose (Adho Mukha Svanasana).*

Figure 2.36. *Type P: Seated forward bend pose (Paschimottanasana).*

Similarly, when performing a backward bend, it is difficult for a Type P to establish the lumbar backward bend, as the lumbar extensor is relatively long and weak and the rectus abdominis is short and strong. Likewise, hip extension will usually take over, as the gluteus maximus can work significantly harder than the psoas.

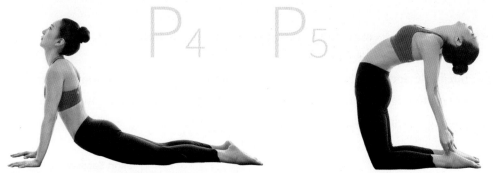

Figure 2.37. *Type P: Upward-facing dog pose (Urdhva Mukha Svanasana).*

Figure 2.38. *Type P: Camel pose (Ustrasana).*

A hip joint extension-oriented backward bend will therefore occur habitually in the Upward-facing dog pose (Figure 2.37) or the Camel pose (Figure 2.38). The tailbone will move downward, whereas the pubic bones will move upward. Such excessive hip extension and contraction of the strong, yet shortened, rectus abdominis will usually prevent the extension of the lumbar vertebrae.

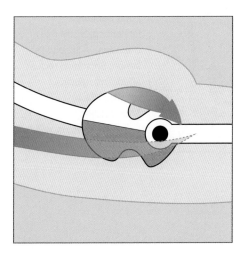
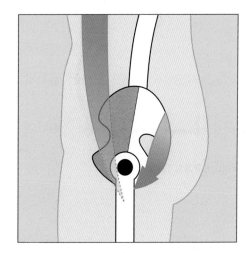

Figure 2.39. *At the front, the rectus abdominis is short and strong (locked-short), while at the back, the gluteus maximus is short and strong (locked-short).*

Both the lumbar area and the hip joint are required to work in unison during the backward bend. In Type P, however, it is mostly the hip joint that is active and lumbar extension is ignored. If such unbalanced backward bends are repeatedly performed and the hip joint is overused, the effect will be to exacerbate an already unbalanced posterior pelvic tilt (PPT).

Section imbalance = connecting spine, pelvis and muscle imbalances.

In Figures 2.40 and 2.41, images of the sections of the body are shown on the left; the diagrams on the right depict a diagnostic analysis of the corresponding musculoskeletal imbalances in the left images.

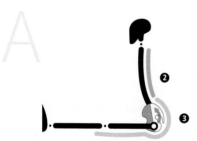
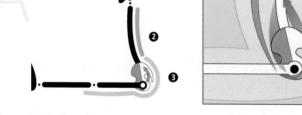

Short Section 2
Anterior pelvic tilt (hip flexion) + lumbar extension. Shortened psoas, erector spinae (blue).
Long Section 3
Lengthened gluteus maximus, rectus abdominis (red).

Figure 2.40. *Type A.*

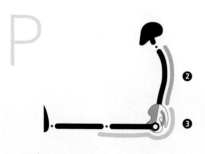
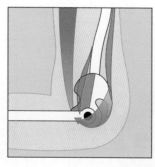

Long Section 2
Posterior pelvic tilt (hip extension) + lumbar flexion. Shortened rectus abdominis, gluteus maximus (blue).
Short Section 3
Lengthened psoas, erector spinae (red).

Figure 2.41. *Type P.*

We can see that, if it is difficult to lengthen Section 3 of the back line and only Section 2 is lengthened during the forward bend, flexion mainly happens at the lumbar joints but not at the hip joint, and that the hamstrings and gluteus maximus in Section 3 are short and the erector spinae in Section 2 are weak. Comparing the visuals on the left and right sides, we can understand the imbalance in joint movement.

Once an understanding of the connection between the section imbalances, joint imbalances, and core muscle imbalances is established, one will be able to start identifying various unbalanced postural types.

"*The one who has found his or her own path in life can truly sympathize with the paths of others. The one who has figured out his or her own imbalances can truly sympathize with and appreciate the imbalances of others.*"

PART II

POSTURAL TYPES

3

Four Postural Types

• • • • • •

P, who is in her early forties, started yoga class with her friend A last month. She was confident that her yoga practice would be nice and easy, as she had been active since childhood and followed a regular exercise regime, favoring mountain climbing. However, P's confidence was crushed in the first class. For one hour, the numerous repeated range of forward bend poses (even the names are difficult to comprehend) gave her a hard time. While it was challenging for P to touch her toes, her friend A could grab her ankles easily within two weeks. P tried her very best, but the more effort she put in, the more the pain at the backs of her thighs increased as her hamstrings stretched further. Her friend enjoyed yoga so much, she suggested P to register for another three months with her. However, P was not sure if yoga asana practice was the right pursuit for her.

After a consultation with the director of the yoga center, P decided to join her friend A and registered for another three months. The key factor that influenced P's decision to continue yoga practice was the realization that she had a certain "body type," aka "postural type." As a result of the consultation, she understood that the reason for her difficulties in forward bends was her excessive posterior pelvic tilt and flat lumbar curvature. Although she had done many kinds of exercises, she had done nothing to correct her slightly hunched body type. After hearing that restoring balance in the core muscles (which are critical for the healthy functioning of the lumbar spine and pelvis) is one of the important aims of yoga asanas, she was certain that this was what she needed.

Her friend A had the opposite body or postural type. A had a strong anterior pelvic tilt and lumbar lordosis, which made it easy for her to perform hip flexion and forward bending poses. However, as the erector spinae muscles of this postural type tend to contract easily, back pain frequently occurs. She found the fundamental solution through yoga after learning the cause of her back pain.

C, who is in her mid-thirties, is a corporate professional. She has been practicing yoga for three years. Six months ago, she started a yoga teacher training course. When she first started yoga practice, most of the poses were not demanding for her and she felt that she had an aptitude for it. However, during the teacher training, she started to face difficulties in some of the advanced poses, such as the Sleeping tortoise. Eventually, she developed back pain, as she drove herself to improve. She indeed improved after two to three weeks, but her back pain returned when she forced herself to overcome new challenges. After three repeated occurrences of the back pain, C started to wonder if she would ever be able to do any advanced yoga asanas.

The difficulties experienced by our heroines A, P, and C can be resolved if we understand their daily postural patterns. Unbalanced postural patterns are not just problems unique to A, P, and C, but a common phenomenon.

Once we know the cause of the problem, we can identify the solution and appropriate a corrective approach. This will make it so much easier for beginners like P. In addition, once Types A and C understand their own imbalances in their core muscles, both the trainer and the trainee will be confident and able to focus on corrective practices.

Differentiating Between Type A and Type P Spinal Curvature and Pelvic Tilt

Type A exhibits the pattern of excessive lumbar lordosis and anterior pelvic tilt; Type P exhibits the pattern of excessive thoracic kyphosis and posterior pelvic tilt (Figure 3.1).

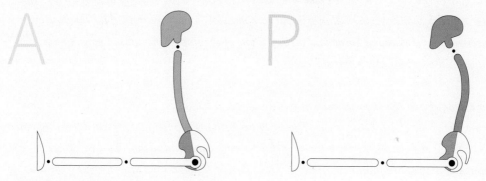

Figure 3.1. *Type A and Type P patterns.*

Sectional Imbalances

We can differentiate between Type A and Type P by focusing on Sections 2 and 3 of the forward and backward bending poses.

Forward Bending Poses

Type A's Section 2 of the back line is short, while Section 3 is long. Type P's Section 2 of the back line is long, while Section 3 is short.

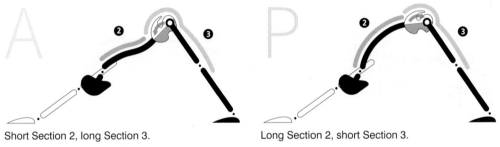

Short Section 2, long Section 3.   Long Section 2, short Section 3.

Figure 3.2. *Forward bending pose—back line patterns.*

Backward Bending Poses

Type A's Section 2 of the front line is long, while Section 3 is short. Type P's Section 2 of the front line is short, while Section 3 is long.

Breathing Patterns

The *inhalation* pattern is more dominant for Type A, while the *exhalation* pattern is more dominant for Type P.

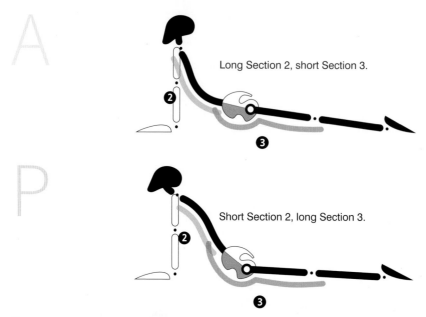

Long Section 2, short Section 3.

Short Section 2, long Section 3.

Figure 3.3. *Backward bending pose—front line patterns.*

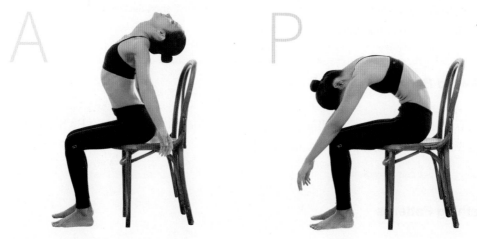

Figure 3.4. *Inhalation and exhalation patterns.*

Comparison of the Forward Bends of Types A and P

Type A's forward bends are more hip joint oriented than lumbar oriented.

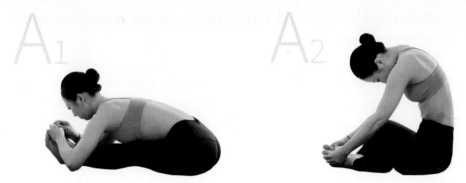

Figure 3.5. *Type A forward bend patterns. Left: Seated forward bend asana (Paschimottanasana)—hip joint forward bend. Right: Bound angle asana (Baddha Konasana) B—lumbar forward bend.*

When Type A does a forward bend, the hip joints can flex well but not the lumbar region; this is illustrated in Figure 3.5—the Seated forward bend pose, which "takes advantage" of the well-facilitated flexion of the hip joint. On the other hand, in the case of the Bound angle pose B (Figure 3.5), which focuses on the lumbar flexion, Type A has much difficulty in executing this.

Type P's forward bends are more lumbar oriented than hip joint oriented.

During a forward bend, Type P tends to flex the lumbar spine efficiently, but not the hip joints; this is illustrated in Figure 3.6, where the multi-section Seated forward bend proves challenging for the hip joints. In contrast, the flexible lumbar region makes the Bound angle pose much more accessible.

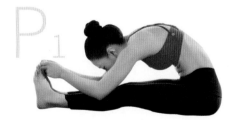
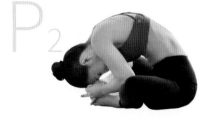

Figure 3.6. *Type P forward bend patterns. Left: Seated forward bend asana (Paschimottanasana)—hip joint forward bend. Right: Bound angle asana (Baddha Konasana) B—lumbar forward bend.*

Due to the imbalances in the core muscles, these unbalanced joint movements become habitual and are repeated subconsciously.

For instance, the pattern of unbalanced joint movement will constantly appear in the Downward-facing dog pose. Type A in Figure 3.7 demonstrates an unbalanced hip-oriented flexion with lumbar extension and anterior pelvic tilt. Type P in Figure 3.7 demonstrates an unbalanced lumbar-oriented flexion and posterior pelvic tilt.

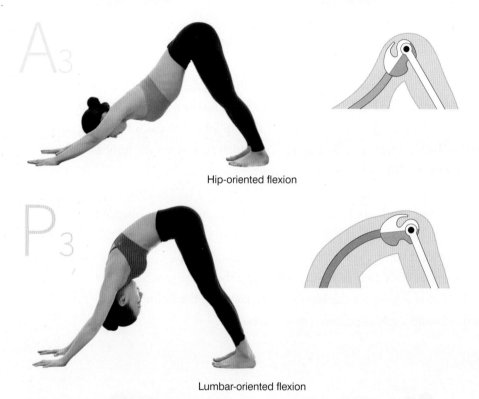

Hip-oriented flexion

Lumbar-oriented flexion

Figure 3.7. *Downward-facing dog pose.*

Comparison of the Backward Bends of Types A and P

For Type A, lumbar extension occurs more naturally in backward bends, while hip joint extension does not. In contrast, for Type P, hip joint extension is spontaneous, but not lumbar extension.

To summarize, Type A mainly uses the hip joints during forward bends and the lumbar region during backward bends. Type P, in contrast, mainly uses the lumbar region during forward bends and the hip joints during backward bends.

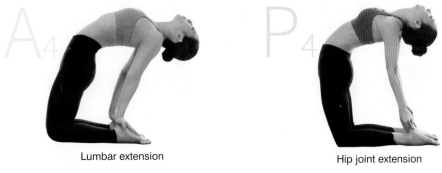

Lumbar extension   Hip joint extension

Figure 3.8. *Camel pose (Ustrasana).*

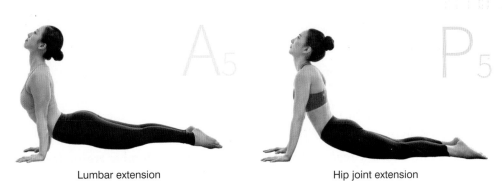

Lumbar extension   Hip joint extension

Figure 3.9. *Upward-facing dog pose (Urdhva Mukha Svanasana).*

Differentiating Between Types A and C

Although both Types A and C have anterior pelvic tilt imbalances, the shapes of their spine curvatures are different, the main differentiator being in the sub-parts (regions) of Section 2.

In Type A, the secondary curvature of the lumbar spine (lordotic) is profound but the primary curvature of the thoracic vertebrae is not.

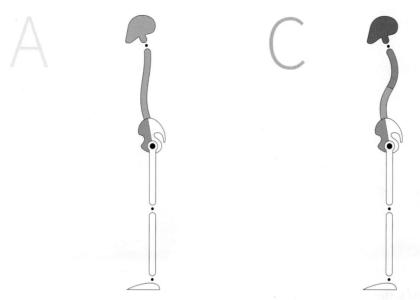

Figure 3.10. *Curvatures of the spine for Types A and C.*

In Type C, the secondary curvature of the lumbar spine is profound and the primary curvature of the thoracic vertebrae is also profound. Type C's lumbar curve is similar to that of Type A, and their thoracic curve is similar to that of Type P.

Spine curvature: the spine of Type A forms a slight C shape and the Type C spine forms an S shape. In the case of Type A, the entire Section 2 of the back line is short. **In Type C, the thoracic region of Section 2 is long and the lumbar region is short**.

Let us look at the forward and backward bends of Types A and C.

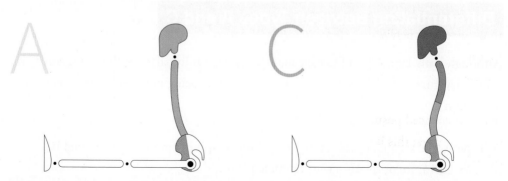

Figure 3.11. *Section 2 shapes for Types A and C in a seated position with straight legs.*

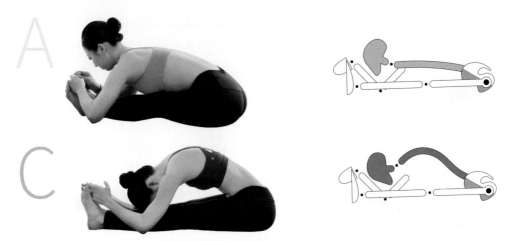

Figure 3.12. *Seated forward bend (Paschimottanasana).*

In forward bends, the lumbar spine appears to be straight and short in both Types A and C. However, the thoracic vertebrae region of the back of Type C appears to be excessively hunched and long.

Types A and C can perform lumbar extension well, but extension of the thoracic vertebrae is difficult for Type C because of excessive kyphosis.

Hip joint extension tends to be difficult for both Types A and C during backward bends. Type A can extend well both the thoracic vertebrae and the lumbar region; however, thoracic extension is hard for Type C.

Looking at the raised pelvis and lifted tailbone in Figure 3.13, we see that the posterior pelvic tilt, also known as *hip joint extension*, is not properly performed.

Looking at the pelvis, which cannot be pushed forward, and the lifted tailbone in Figure 3.14, we can conclude that the posterior pelvic tilt, also known as *hip joint extension*, is not properly performed.

Such unbalanced postural patterns may not change completely, even after years of practicing yoga; this is because our daily unbalanced postural patterns often repeat subconsciously, even during yoga asana practice and our daily lives.

If the unbalanced joint movement pattern is obvious and also difficult to correct, it is important to identify the associated postural type—the root cause of the imbalances.

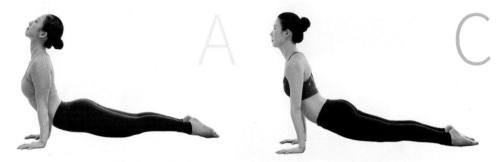

Figure 3.13. *Upward-facing dog pose (Urdhva Mukha Svanasana).*

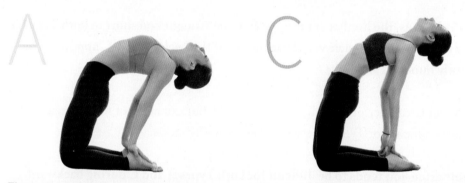

Figure 3.14. *Camel pose (Ustrasana).*

Four Postural Types

Unbalanced postural patterns are formed because of changes in spine curvature and pelvic tilt. These, in turn, are usually caused by imbalances in the hip joints and deep core muscles of the lumbar region.

Imbalances in the deep core muscles → changes to spine curvature and pelvic tilt → unbalanced postural patterns.

It is common for people with unbalanced lumbar and pelvic patterns to have an imbalance in other areas, such as the hip joints, knees, and feet.

There is a connection between all the unbalanced patterns throughout the body. An unbalanced pattern in, for example, the shoulder blades and other joints is linked to the patterns of unbalanced postures and even unbalanced breathing. These combine to form the postural type.

Spinal and pelvic imbalances + lower limb imbalances + upper limb imbalances + breathing imbalances = body type or postural type.

If these patterns are consistently repeated in the different asanas, a wider pattern, comprised of the sub-patterns, can be identified. A set of postural patterns can be called *body type* or *postural type*.

A *postural type* is a combination of breathing and postural patterns, where breathing and patterns of pelvic tilt form the key elements.

Pelvic tilt directly affects the curvature of the spine. Breathing affects the energy patterns and the direction of the rotation of the upper and lower limbs.

Postural type can be divided into four main elements:

1. Pelvic tilt
2. Spinal curvature
3. Breathing
4. Energy patterns

After analyzing each of the above elements and observing their repetitive and consistent order of appearance in yoga asana practice, we will be able to identify the postural type.

Type A: Anterior Expansion Type

The strengthening effect of the inhalation pattern on the anterior pelvic tilt and lumbar extension characterize Type A.

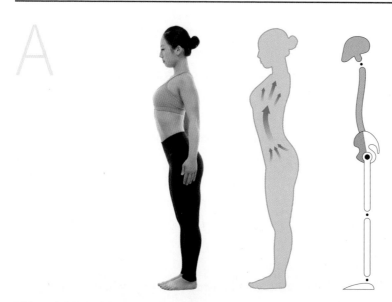

Figure 3.15. *Anterior expansion Type A.*

In Type A, the hip flexors and erector spinae muscles are short and strong, because of the anterior pelvic tilt (APT). On the other hand, the hip extensors and rectus abdominis muscles are long and weak. Lordosis is excessive, the hip joints are internally rotated, and the feet are pronated.

In general, Type A appears to be expanded with an arched back. The C-shape curvature of the lumbar spine is clear and distinct. The chest is open confidently and the shoulders are rolled back. The tailbone is lifted, and the pubic bone moves downward. A closer inspection will reveal an anterior pelvic tilt.

A represents the **a**nterior pelvic tilt and **E** the **e**xpansion of energy, and so for future reference we can call this *Type AE* (or simplified as *Type A*). This type derives from the combination of its most pronounced characteristics of both an anterior pelvic tilt and inhalation-oriented expansion energy patterns.

Type P: Posterior Contraction Type

The strengthening effect of the exhalation pattern on the posterior pelvic tilt and lumbar flexion characterize Type P.

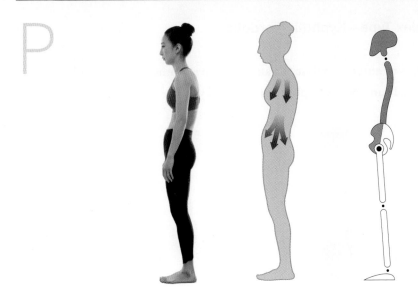

Figure 3.16. *Posterior contraction Type P.*

In Type P, because of posterior pelvic tilt (PPT), the hip extensors and rectus abdominis muscles are short and strong. On the other hand, the hip flexors and erector spinae muscles are long and weak. Thoracic kyphosis is excessive. External rotation of the hip joint and a supination pattern of the feet are evident.

In general, Type P appears to be contracted and bent inward. The lumbar spine is flat, while the upper back appears to be stooped. The chest seems to be curved in and the shoulders are rolled in. The tailbone is dropped and the pubic bone moves upward. A closer inspection will reveal a posterior pelvic tilt.

P represents the **p**osterior pelvic tilt and **C** the **c**ontraction of energy, and so it can be called *Type PC* (or simply *Type P*). This type derives from the combination of its most pronounced characteristics of both a posterior pelvic tilt and an inward contraction of energy.

Type AE (anterior expansion) and Type PC (posterior contraction) will manifest naturally in the pelvic tilt and the breathing pattern. As the characteristics of the patterns are clear and distinct, they will be relatively easy to recognize.

Type C, described next, is not as easy to identify.

Type C: Complex Type—Kyphotic-Lordotic

The characteristics of anterior pelvic tilt and excessive lumbar lordosis and thoracic kyphosis can all be found in the kyphotic-lordotic Type C.

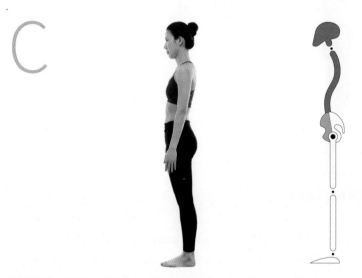

Figure 3.17. *Kyphotic-lordotic Type C.*

In Type C, the hip flexors and erector spinae muscles are short and strong. The anterior pelvic tilt pattern is obvious. However, the hip joints rotate internally and the feet are usually pronated. Careful observation and judgment are required, as the lumbar region and pelvis behave as Type A, while the thoracic region behaves as Type P.

Type C (**c**omplex type) is complicated and both the practitioner and the observer may struggle to distinguish this type. There is a lumbar lordosis and an anterior pelvic tilt, similar to Type A, but it is usually more pronounced; moreover, there is a thoracic kyphosis with protracted shoulder blades and internal rotation of the shoulder joints, as in Type P.

When the lumbar and limb patterns are similar to Type A, but the thoracic vertebrae and upper limbs are similar to Type P, this indicates Type C. It is important to emphasize here, however, that Type C is difficult to diagnose correctly.

Type N: Neutral Type

A neutral pelvis, well-balanced curvature of the lumbar and thoracic vertebrae, neutral rotation of the hip joints, and neutral position of the feet are characteristics of Type N.

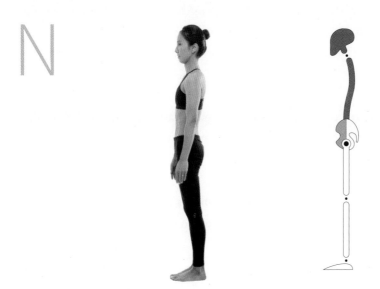

Figure 3.18. *Neutral Type N.*

Three Major Patterns: Pelvic Tilt, Spinal Curvature, Breathing Energy

Pattern	Type AE (anterior expansion type)	Type PC (posterior contraction type)	Type C (complex type)	Type N (neutral type)
Pelvic tilt	Anterior pelvic tilt (APT)	Posterior pelvic tilt (PPT)	Anterior pelvic tilt (APT)	Neutral pelvis (neutral)
Spinal curvature	Lordosis	Kyphosis	Kyphotic-lordotic	Balanced
Breathing energy	Inhalation and expansion	Exhalation and contraction	Mixed	Balanced

Figure 3.19. *Patterns and body types.*

Spinopelvic Imbalances and Lower Limb Movement Patterns

Unbalanced patterns of the spine and pelvis can affect the direction of the movement of the limb joints.

If the hip joints are flexed when the pelvis bends forward (anterior tilt) in the upright position, the internal rotators of the hips work smoothly. As a result, internal rotation of the entire leg and pronation of the feet occur effortlessly as the hip joints rotate internally.

When extending the hip in a posterior tilt, the external rotating muscles of the hip will readily activate. As a result, external rotation of the hip joints and supination of the feet follow naturally.

In summary, anterior pelvic tilt (hip flexion) contributes to internal hip rotation, while posterior pelvic tilt (hip extension) contributes to external hip rotation.

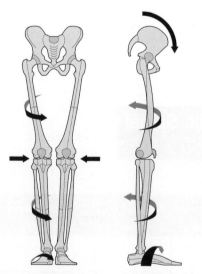 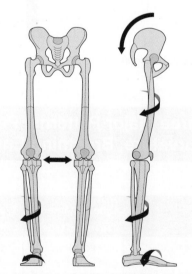

Left two images: anterior pelvic tilt, internal rotation of the hip joint, internal rotation of the tibia, and pronation of the foot.

Right two images: posterior pelvic tilt, external rotation of the hip joint, external rotation of the tibia, and supination of the foot.

Figure 3.20. *Impact of pelvic imbalances on the lower limbs.*

If the relation between an unbalanced anterior/posterior pelvic tilt and an internal/external rotation of the leg is understood, one can then understand and guesstimate unbalanced internal/external rotation patterns of the limbs in Type A, P, and C.

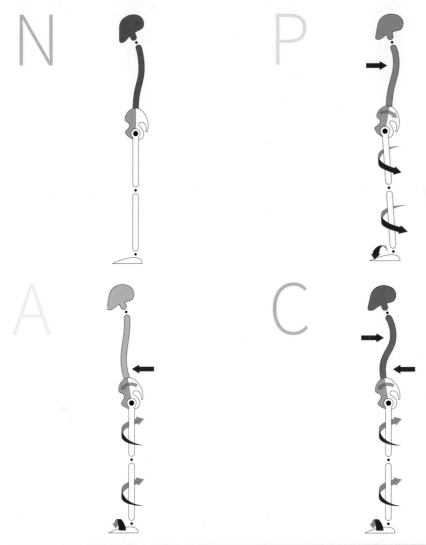

Region	Type N Neutral	Type A Anterior	Type P Posterior	Type C Complex
Spine	Balanced	Lumbar lordosis	Thoracic kyphosis	Thoracic kyphosis, lumbar lordosis
Pelvic tilt	Neutral pelvis	Anterior	Posterior	Anterior
Hip joint	Neutral	Internal rotation	External rotation	Internal rotation
Tibia	Neutral	Internal rotation	External rotation	Internal rotation
Foot	Neutral	Pronation	Supination	Pronation

Figure 3.21. *All types and patterns.*

4

The Dilemma of Imbalance

Imbalances in the upright standing position are a unique feature of humans, in contrast to quadrupedal animals. It has taken the human species about seven million years to evolve to a biped. Now, we complete our physical development in the course of about 15 years. Millions of years of evolution have made an unconscious imprint on our physique, implanting various unbalanced postural patterns, which are presented in this book as postural Types A, P, and C.

Yoga was developed over 3000 years by countless generations of people; it aims to achieve a balance of the mind through the balance of posture and breathing. A balanced breathing pattern is essential for a balanced mind. Unbalanced breathing leads to imbalances in the autonomic nervous system—something that is very common in the population. In addition, postural balance is essential, as it is strongly related to breathing patterns.

The Dilemma of the Upright Position: Beginning of Imbalance

The human fetus floats like a fish inside its mother's womb. After birth, the baby lies flat on the ground like a snake and then crawls like a dog, starting to explore walking at the age of one. Just like a frog, not being able to recall its tadpole days, most people cannot remember this process at all. Standing upright and walking are unconscious patterns of learning rather than our inborn abilities.

A person's shift toward bipedalism is normally completed by about 15 years of age, when the efficiency of burning calories for bipedalism is similar to that of an adult.

While a modern human's upright development begins at about one year of age and is accomplished by the age of 15 years, mankind's evolution to an upright being started seven million years ago and was completed about 150,000 years ago. The early archeoanthropine sahelanthropus tchadensis, which were discovered in Chad, Africa, were fully developed into the homo sapiens stage just 150,000 years ago. (See *Human Locomotion* by Thomas C. Michaud.*)

Everyone carries postural imbalances, without realizing that this is an outcome of seven million years of evolution to a biped rather than just 15 years of a single human being's development.

Although humans have derived great benefit from the upright position in terms of freedom of hands, wide vision, language, and developed brain, we must also deal with the imbalances that come with the unstable bipedal position.

It takes time and effort to understand the fact that we are all unbalanced bipeds. This conscious training of restoring the balance is a lifetime complex process.

It is not easy to stand in a perfectly balanced upright position. If one opens the chest, the buttocks will be pushed out. If the buttocks are lowered, the back will be stooped. If the chest is opened, the tailbone will be lifted by the excessive lumbar curvature. If the tailbone is rolled down, the abdomen will be pushed out and the thoracic curvature will become more pronounced.

*Michaud, T.C. 2011. *Human Locomotion: The Conservative Management of Gait-related Disorders*, Newton Biomechanics: Newton, MA, USA.

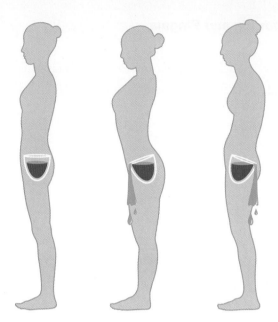

Figure 4.1. *Models in an upright standing position: (left to right) balanced, anterior pelvic tilt, and posterior pelvic tilt.*

Anterior pelvic tilt (middle model in Figure 4.1) illustrates the increase in lumbar curvature, similar to the spilling of the water. This posture leads to the loss of energy (metaphorically water) because of the increase in consumption.

Sticking with the water-spilling metaphor, if the pelvis tilts posteriorly and the lumbar curvature diminishes (right model in Figure 4.1), water will spill backward—an underproduction of energy will therefore occur.

A lot of people, more than we imagine, are experiencing such upright postural difficulties.

There are two types of upright postural dilemma, which are closely related to both the external appearance and the state of mind.

Energy Channel for Ida and Pingala

The unbalanced energy model, called *Ida and Pingala* in Hatha Yoga, could explain the cause of a postural dilemma from the energy standpoint (Pranamaya Kosha).

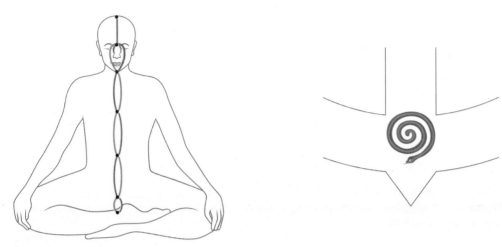

Figure 4.2. *Central channel (Sushumna) and coiled serpent (Kundalini).*

A coiled serpent (Kundalini) blocks the way to physical and energetic balance. When the way to Sushumna (central neutral channel) is purified and opened through the practices (tapas), one will be able to break free from the postural dilemma and achieve a balance. (See *Yoga Taravali* for a detailed explanation.*)

There is a connection between the physical basis of the postural quest and energy imbalances of the human attitude—optimism vs. pessimism, activity vs. passivity, aggression vs. defensiveness, masculinity vs. femininity, etc.

The physical posture is an external expression of the attitude of the mind. Conversely, the attitude of the mind is an internal expression of the posture.

According to Hatha yoga's systematic method, to change your attitude you first need to change your posture; this will lead to an improved state of mind. Yoga postures are a good start toward approaching balance, starting with the body and progressing to the mind.

---

*Desikachar, T.K.V. and Desikachar, K. 2003. *Adi Sankara's Yoga Taravali*, Krishnamacharya Yoga Mandiram: India.

Unbalanced Postural and Breathing Patterns

Postural patterns affect breathing patterns, and vice versa. When the chest is open, both anterior pelvic tilt and lumbar curvature (secondary curvature) increase; this is called the *inhalation pattern*, as it is a postural pattern formed by a deep inhalation.

If you roll in the tailbone, both posterior pelvic tilt and thoracic curvature (primary curvature) increase; this is called the *exhalation pattern*, as it is a postural pattern formed by a deep exhalation.

The front line of Section 2 is lengthened during inhalation, while the back line of Section 2 is lengthened during exhalation.

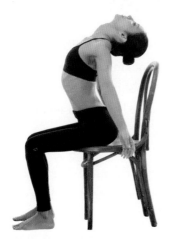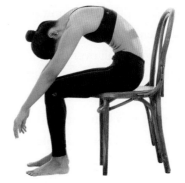

Figure 4.3. *Inhalation and exhalation patterns.*

A Type A, with a more prominent inhalation pattern, will likely have an unconsciously weak exhalation pattern. On the contrary, a Type P, with a more prominent exhalation pattern, will have weak inhalation patterns.

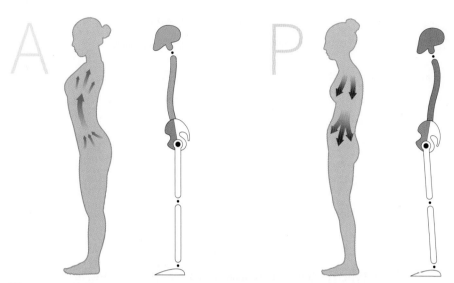

Figure 4.4. *Models showing inhalation (A) and exhalation (P) patterns.*

Generally, it is difficult for people to recognize their own posture objectively, because they usually only see the front part of their body when looking in the mirror. People can feel their posture through proprioceptors, such as the skin or vestibular system, which are spread all over the body. However, if the posture becomes a lifelong habit, which is hard to mend, it is challenging to feel it.

To quote Agatha Christie, "Curious things, habits. People themselves never knew they had them." Even if people can recognize their postural patterns by looking in a mirror or at a video, or through the feedback from others, it is very difficult to receive "live" updates on their patterns during everyday life and make attempts to correct the imbalances.

Constantly adjusting posture and breath to form new habits is a complicated task to maintain. Although people will try poses that are more beneficial for their posture, it is not easy to consistently combine these poses with the corrective breathing rhythm, and often tension arises unconsciously.

For example, in the case of Type A, where the inhalation pattern of expanding the chest and raising the tailbone is fixed, as one exhales, one needs to combine the exhalation pattern consciously, where the tailbone is rolled in and the jaw is pulled down.

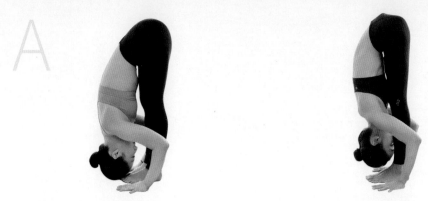

Figure 4.5. *Type A before correction (left). Correction toward neutral by tucking in the jaw and rolling in the tailbone during exhalation (right).*

On the other hand, for Type P, where the exhalation pattern is dominant, one can aim toward neutral by emphasizing the opposite patterns, such as expanding the chest and raising the tailbone consciously during inhalation.

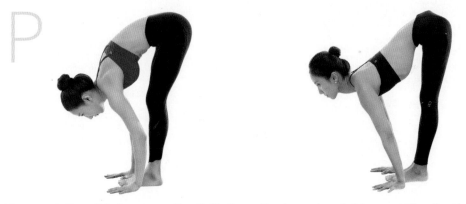

Figure 4.6. *Type P before correction (left). Correction toward neutral by expanding the chest and raising the tailbone during inhalation (right).*

The conscious effort of bringing the postural inhalation pattern into the fixed exhalation pattern, as well as bringing the postural exhalation pattern into the fixed inhalation pattern, is a good start in achieving a balanced posture.

"'1% theory and 99% practice' is the key to making 1% of seed sprout from 99% of the fallen fruit."

PART III

ADJUSTMENTS

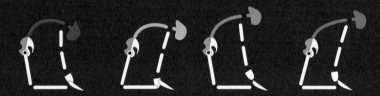

5

Strategies and Goals for Correcting Imbalances

• • • • • •

I n Chapters 5–8 of Part III, we will learn corrective methods for restoring a
neutral position of the pelvis and the spinal curvature for Types A, P, and C. I will
subsequently explain traditional techniques for limb alignment, spinal balance, and
breath control in Chapters 9 and 10.

If you have identified your body type (the best technique is through observation of
your patterns in a small group of yoga practitioners), you should first look for the
corrective methods in Chapters 5–8, and only then practice the techniques of limb
alignment and breathing, presented in Chapters 9 and 10.

Relationship between posture and breathing	• Spinal balance breathing control
	• Chapter 10
Relationship between torso and limbs	• Alignment of limbs
	• Chapter 9
Relationship between spine and pelvis	• Correction according to body type
	• Chapters 6–8

Figure 5.1. *Relationship chart: posture and breathing, torso and limbs, and spine and pelvis.*

Specific Correction Goals for Different Body Types

The basic aim of a forward bend is to lengthen the back line of the body through the
flexion of the hip joints and lumbar vertebrae. The fundamental purpose of a backward
bend is to lengthen the front line of the body through the extension of the hip joints
and lumbar vertebrae.

People of Type N, who do not have excessive sectional imbalances, will not experience much difficulty in either forward or backward bends during yoga practice.

However, people of Types A, P, and C, who have significant sectional imbalances in the spinal and pelvic regions, will experience a worsening in the unbalanced movement of specific joints during forward or backward bends, as shown in Part I (observation) and Part II (postural types). The basic intention of lengthening the back and front line of the body may be distorted, resulting in a worsening of the sectional imbalances.

The imbalance of the lumbar and hip joints therefore needs to be correctly identified, on the basis of the body/postural type. Through further corrective practice, **the neutral position of pelvic tilt and the balance of spinal curvature can be restored**.

The goal is not simply to lengthen the front and back lines of the body, but, first, to establish clear objectives, on the basis of the postural type, and only then to develop a strategy and devise a corrective method.

Specific Aims for the Different Body Types

Type A: lengthening Section 2 of the back line and lengthening Section 3 of the front line. Restoring balance through posterior pelvic tilt movement and lumbar flexion.

Type P: lengthening Section 3 of the back line and lengthening Section 2 of the front line. Restoring balance through anterior pelvic tilt movement and lumbar extension.

Type C: lengthening Section 2 of the back line in the lumbar region, lengthening Section 2 of the front line in the chest region, and lengthening Section 3 of the front line. Restoring balance through posterior pelvic tilt movement, lumbar flexion, and thoracic extension.

Correction Strategies for the Different Body Types

To restore the neutral position of the pelvis, Types A and C need to tilt their pelvis posteriorly, while Type P needs to tilt their pelvis anteriorly. However, in most multi-section postures, movement of the pelvis is often limited because of the tension in the unbalanced muscles in Sections 2 and 3. Therefore, for an effective correction, a temporary loosening of the tension in the pelvis and spine in Sections 2 and 3 is required.

One effective method to use in forward bends is a slight bend in the knees, which enables a temporary freedom of the pelvic movement. Having the knees bent reduces the muscle tension between Sections 3 and 4, and makes a posterior pelvic tilt easier for Types A and C. If the conditions for an easier posterior pelvic tilt are provided, Section 2 of the back line can be effectively lengthened through lumbar flexion, which is the primary corrective cue for forward bends of Type A. Type C can also effectively achieve the primary and secondary goals, which are lumbar flexion and thoracic extension respectively, by bending the knees.

In addition, it is easier for Type P to perform an anterior pelvic tilt if the knees are slightly bent. If the conditions for easier anterior pelvic tilt are provided, Section 3 of the back line can be effectively lengthened through hip flexion, which is the primary corrective goal for forward bends for Type P.

For backward bends with all body types, restoring balance between pelvic tilt and lumbar extension is the key point.

In the case of Type A, where posterior pelvic tilt movement is limited, this can be aided through conscious use of the gluteal muscles. Section 3 of the front line can then be effectively lengthened through extension of the hip joint, which is the primary corrective goal for Type A.

Type C should also seek to facilitate hip joint extension and posterior pelvic tilt by intentionally engaging the gluteal muscles. This should be followed by thoracic extension, which is the secondary goal for Type C.

For Type P, as the hip extensors of the gluteal muscles are already over-activated, the tension in the gluteal muscles should be reduced and the erector spinae muscles can be contracted, while extending the lumbar and thoracic vertebrae. This way, Type P can achieve their primary goal of lengthening Section 2 of the front line.

Q2 What Is the Standard for Balance and Imbalance?

Movement of the body can be analyzed on the basis of the direction of the movements of the joints. In order to define the direction of joint movement, a base standard is required. For this you need to view the body in a neutral position, in which all joints are in a neutral state. An example of such a position is Samasthiti pose. In functional anatomy, we would say that a body in Samasthiti is in the anatomical position.

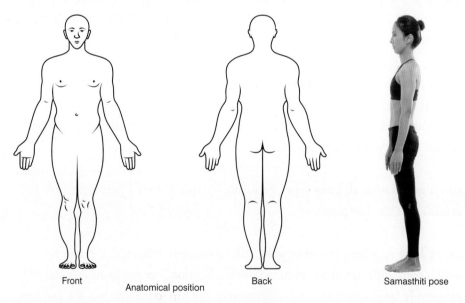

Front
Back
Samasthiti pose

Anatomical position

Figure 5.2. *Anatomical position and Samasthiti pose.*

In relation to the anatomical position:

- Movement of the body and limbs toward the front is known as *flexion*.
- Movement toward the back is known as *extension*.
- The various types of joint movement are flexion, extension, adduction, abduction, and internal and external rotation.

Samasthiti is a posture that requires an equal and steady stance in all directions; *Sama* means "equal" and *Sthit* means "to establish."

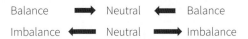

Balance is a state that is as close to neutral as possible, while *imbalance* refers to a state that is further away from neutral.

A good start toward reaching balance is to develop an awareness of your own unbalanced states, rather than attempting to use other people's bodies as a reference point. If you can identify the imbalance correctly, you will be able to find a way to rectify it.

If a practitioner's upright posture is not neutral and already in a state of imbalance, this will be reflected in all other movements. Forward, backward, and sideways bends and twisting poses will also become unbalanced.

Observation of the effects of an unbalanced upright position on asana patterns is therefore a key element of intelligent yoga practice.

Q3 People Commonly Think That Improving Flexibility is the Goal of Yoga Practice, but According to This Book, the Goal of Asana Practice Is Restoring Balance. If So, How Will Flexibility Help in Restoring Balance?

According to the Yoga Sutras of Patanjali, a yoga posture (asana) should be easy/comfortable (sukha) and steady/stable (sthira).

First, for a posture to be easy/comfortable (sukha), there should be no restrictions in the movements of the joints; any restriction at the joints will lead to discomfort. If flexibility of the joints is limited, postural imbalances will occur and it will be difficult to correct them. Therefore, people may think that yoga postures only focus on improving flexibility.

But if a person is just flexible and not steady/stable (sthira) at the joints, this will also result in imbalances. Practice should therefore combine flexibility and steadiness or stability.

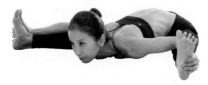

Figure 5.3. *Wide-angle seated forward bend A (Upavistha Konasana A).*

For instance, in the Wide-angle seated forward bend (Upavistha Konasana), where the joints are moving away from the mid-line in abduction, it is more important to reach the feet with the hands and maintain a strong abduction angle, rather than opening a hip joint angle wider. Reaching the feet will stabilize the joints, providing support for such an intense stretch.

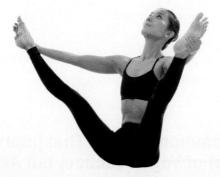

Figure 5.4. *Wide-angle seated forward bend B (Upavistha Konasana B).*

In the Wide-angle seated forward bend B, where the legs are raised and the entire body rests on the sit bones, the main goal is to improve stability through the balance of adduction and abduction in this abduction-centric state.

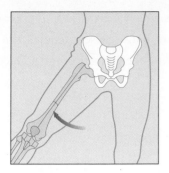 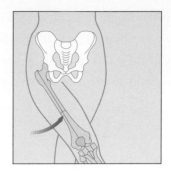

Figure 5.5. *Hip joint abduction (left image) and adduction (right image).*

In the coronal plane, which divides the body into front and back parts, *abduction of the hip* means movement away from the mid-line of the body. On the other hand, *adduction of the hip* refers to movement toward the mid-line of the body.

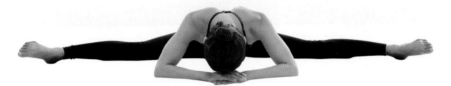

Figure 5.6. *Forward bend in straight angle pose.*

As shown in Figure 5.6, if one focuses only on stretching in the abduction direction, the flexibility of the joints toward the abduction will improve, but the strength for the counteraction toward the adduction will diminish. Eventually, the stability between adduction and abduction of the joints will be lost. The abductors will become shortened (locked-short) because of overuse, while the adductors will lose their strength (locked-long).

The Samakonasana pose, illustrated in Figure 5.7, is an advanced asana, not because it is just a flexibility pose that stretches the adductors, but because it requires the stability of the joints to be maintained while balancing the abduction and adduction movements in an extreme abduction pose.

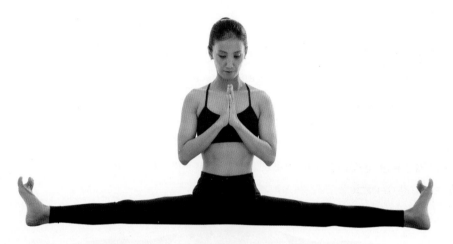

Figure 5.7. *Straight angle pose (Samakonasana).*

If one focuses just on flexibility, the joint movement will be disproportionate in one direction. Regardless of whether or not this is a conscious action, the result will be hyperflexion or hyperextension, hyperabduction or hyperadduction, hyper-external rotation or hyper-internal rotation, and so on and so forth.

A balance between flexion and extension, abduction and adduction, and external and internal rotation can be achieved through conscious practice and corrective actions that focus on both flexibility and stability.

Yoga Sutra II-46: sthira sukham asanam

"An asana should be steady and easy or comfortable"

6

Adjustments for Type P

• • • • • •

The purpose of the adjustments for Type P is to counteract the sectional imbalances.

You will recall from Chapter 3 that Type P has an exaggerated posterior pelvic tilt and thoracic kyphosis; the hip extensors and rectus abdominis are strong, whereas the hip flexors and erector spinae muscles are weak. This type is also characterized by the inward contraction of energy.

To counteract sectional imbalances, Section 3 of the back line can be lengthened through forward bends, while Section 2 of the front line can be lengthened through backward bends.

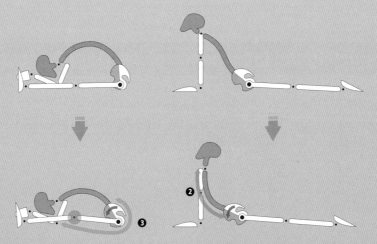

Figure 6.1. *Type P: counteracting the imbalances of the front and back lines.*

Restoring the Direction of Joint Movements

In Type P, hip flexion and lumbar extension are not fully activated, because of long and weak psoas and erector spinae muscles. Type P should therefore strengthen the hip flexor and lumbar extensors.

The left image of Figure 6.2 illustrates the imbalance of Type P; for comparison purposes, the right image shows the opposite pattern of Type A.

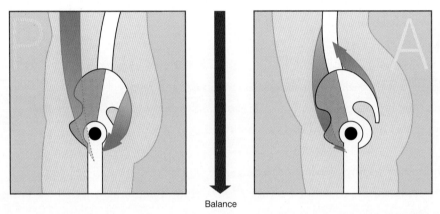

Balance

Figure 6.2. *Type P: Short and strong muscles: rectus abdominis and gluteus maximus (blue). Type A: Short and strong muscles: psoas and erector spinae (blue).*

Counteracting the Imbalances of the Core Muscles

When the psoas is awakened, the gluteus maximus muscle lengthens; similarly, when the erector spinae muscles are strengthened, the rectus abdominis muscle lengthens.

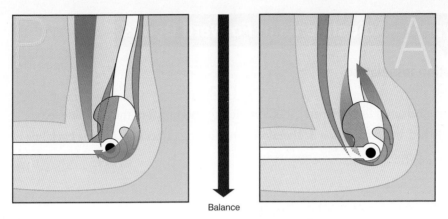

Figure 6.3.
Type P:
Blue: strong *rectus abdominis, gluteus maximus.*
Red: weak *psoas, erector spinae.*

Type A:
Blue: strong *psoas, erector spinae.*
Red: weak *rectus abdominis, gluteus maximus.*

Reversing the Imbalance in Breathing

Induce a balance between inhalation and exhalation by focusing more on the inhalation pattern.

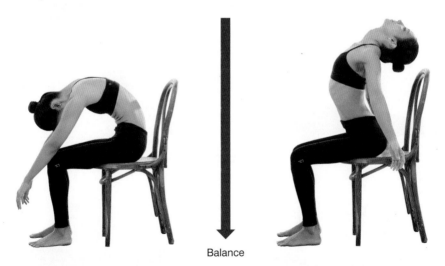

Figure 6.4. *Exhalation pattern and Inhalation pattern.*

Type P—Adjustments in Forward Bends

Section Imbalance

In an unbalanced forward bend, it is common for Section 2 of the back line to be lengthened, but not Section 3. Therefore, lengthening of Section 3 of the back line is the primary purpose of any adjustments.

Unbalanced Lumbopelvic Rhythm

Lumbar flexion is easier for Type P than hip flexion. The use of props will help beginners to facilitate more hip flexion.

Poses such as Bound angle B, a forward bend that focuses on the lumbar area, do not require much effort; however, poses such as Downward-facing dog and seated forward bends, which focus on the hip joints, are relatively difficult for Type P.

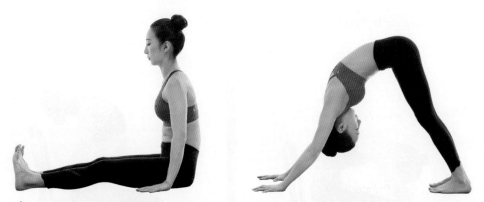

Figure 6.5. *Staff pose (Dandasana). Downward-facing dog pose (Adho MukhaSvanasana).*

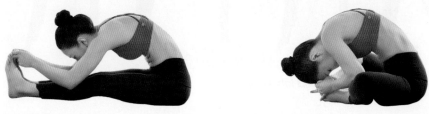

Figure 6.6. *Seated forward bend pose (Paschimottanasana). Bound angle pose (Baddha Konasana) B.*

Adjustments for the Seated Forward Bend Pose (Paschimottanasana)

It is difficult for Type P to effectively perform hip flexion, since the agonists—the psoas major muscles—are not fully active, and the antagonists—the gluteus maximus muscles and the hamstrings—are short and strong.

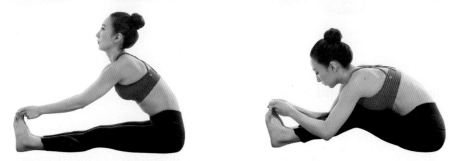

Figure 6.7. *Type P: correct Seated forward bend (Paschimottanasana).*

If a beginner has a posterior pelvic tilt and over-straightens the knees while in a forward bend, this will eventually intensify the lumbar flexion and can lead to back pain or a hamstrings injury.

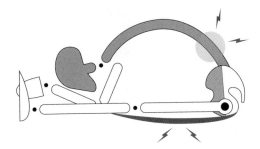

Figure 6.8. *Type P: incorrect Seated forward bend (Paschimottanasana).*

In a Seated forward bend pose, it is therefore wise to either bend the knees or place a bolster underneath the knees to relieve excessive tension in the back line from the lumbar spine to the hamstrings.

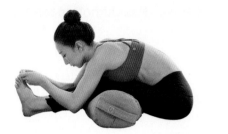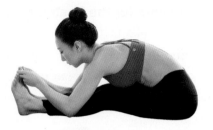

Figure 6.9. *Type P in propped correct Seated forward bend (Paschimottanasana).*

Standing Forward Bend Pose (Uttanasana)

The same logic as for seated forward bends applies to standing forward bends, i.e., bending the knees first to relieve the tension from Section 3 of the back line. Subsequently, an anterior pelvic tilt can be initiated, followed by the gentle and slow action of straightening the knees and then lengthening of Section 3 of the back line.

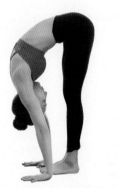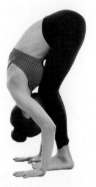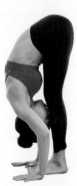

Figure 6.10. *Type P in Standing forward bend pose (Uttanasana).*

Q4 If the Knees Are Bent, Will This Limit the Lengthening of Section 3 of the Back Line?

Let us evaluate this together. The back line of Section 3 is comprised of the thighs and hips. When the hamstrings are stretched, a portion of the thighs is lengthened as well. The origin of the hamstrings is found on the sit bones—the *ischial tuberosities*, while the bones below the knees—the tibias and fibulas—are the sites of the insertion.

In sitting poses, the hamstrings lengthen when the knees are straightened, since the insertion points (tibias, fibulas) move further away. With the knees bent, the hamstrings shorten, because the insertion points move closer.

The hamstrings get longer when the sit bones are further away, because the origins move further away. On the other hand, the hamstrings are shortened when the sit bones are closer, because the origins move closer.

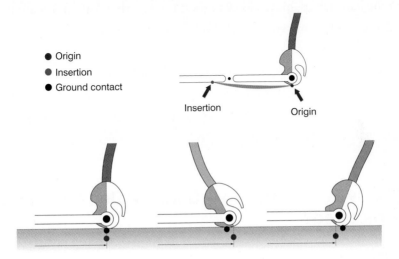

Figure 6.11. *Effects of neutral (left), anterior (center), and posterior (right) pelvic tilt on the origin of the hamstrings.*

As shown in Figure 6.11, when the pelvis tilts anteriorly (center image), the ischial tuberosity (origin, red dot) moves away from the insertion (blue dot), since the origin is displaced backward relative to the ground contact (black dot). In contrast, the ischial tuberosity moves nearer to the insertion when the pelvis tilts posteriorly (right image), because the origin is displaced forward relative to the ground contact.

Within Section 3, the area around the hip is lengthened when the gluteal muscles are lengthened. The gluteal muscles will also be lengthened by an anterior pelvic tilt and shortened by a posterior pelvic tilt accordingly.

In summary, the answer to the question above is "Yes" and "No," because bending the knees limits the lengthening of the thigh but helps in lengthening the hip.

Q5 When the Sit Bones Move Back in an Anterior Pelvic Tilt, the Action of the Lengthening of the Hamstrings and the Gluteal Muscles Is Clear. If the Knees Are Bent, the Hamstrings Contract or Shorten. Does This Not Cancel Out the Effect of the Anterior Pelvic Tilt?

That is correct. If you bend the knees, the tibias and fibulas, which are the "arrival station" of the hamstrings, move closer to the sit bones, the "departure station." This will reduce the lengthening effect caused by the anterior pelvic tilt.

The initial goal of bending the knees and tilting the pelvis anteriorly, however, is not to lengthen the hamstrings; it is rather a preparation for the second stage, where the hamstrings are lengthened from the arrival station (insertion point), when the knees are straightened.

Q6 Why Is a Preparatory Stage of Bending the Knees required?

If the knees are completely straight, there is no free space for the anterior movement of the pelvis. This is because the tensions of the calf muscles (gastrocnemius), in Section 4, and the hamstrings, in Section 3, overlap. By slightly bending the knees, a space is created and the sit bones can move backward by inclining the pelvis anteriorly. This preparation simply releases the effect of the combined tensions in Sections 3 and 4.

Excessive bending of the knees, however, could also limit the lengthening of the hamstrings as they contract. Bending the knees slightly, or putting a cushion of the appropriate height below the knees, can help to loosen the tension and bring the sit bones backward while not shortening the hamstrings too much, thus creating an ideal condition for tilting the pelvis anteriorly more easily.

For Type P, the first stage itself is instrumental. The harder Type P tries to push in a forward bend, the worse the imbalance becomes, as contraction of the rectus abdominis makes the lumbar flexion stronger. This becomes a vicious cycle that interrupts the movement of the anterior pelvic tilt, because excessive posterior pelvic tilt prevents muscles such as psoas from tilting the pelvis anteriorly.

Once the knees are bent slightly and anterior pelvic tilt is facilitated, favorable conditions are created for the erector spinae muscles to overcome the lumbar flexion caused by the abdominal muscles.

At this point, the interaction of the psoas and erector spinae muscles as synergists will become an advantage. Once this stage is reached, the second stage of straightening the knees and lengthening the hamstrings becomes much easier.

The knees, which were bent slightly in the first stage, will require a complete straightening in the second stage for the hamstrings in Section 3 to lengthen fully. It may seem a little complicated, but when it is put into practice, the effects will be immediately apparent and the difference will be obvious.

Type P—Adjustments in Backward Bends

Section Imbalance

In an unbalanced backward bend, it is common to see a lengthening of Section 3 of the front line, but not of Section 2. Lengthening of Section 2 of the front line is therefore the goal of any adjustments.

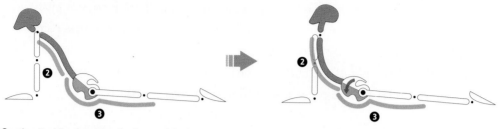

Section 2 of the front line is short, while Section 3 is long. There is difficulty in extending the lumbar and thoracic vertebrae. The hip joints are overextended.

The tailbone needs to lift while the hips are intentionally tilted anteriorly (anterior pelvic tilt). Section 2 of the front line should be lengthened before connecting to Section 3.

Figure 6.12. *Type P in Upward-facing dog pose: before adjustment in the multi-section backward bend (left), and after adjustment (right).*

Unbalanced Lumbopelvic Rhythm

Normally, for Type P, hip extension is easier than lumbar extension. To achieve balanced lumbar extension, corrective methods for lifting and extending the chest and abdomen are necessary.

For Type P, hip joint extension is easier than lumbar extension in poses such as Upward-facing dog, Camel pose, and Upward plank pose. As a result of the strong gluteus maximus muscles and hamstrings, hip joint extension will mainly occur in backward bends. At the same time, because of a relatively strong rectus abdominis and weak erector spinae muscles, it is difficult to achieve lumbar extension.

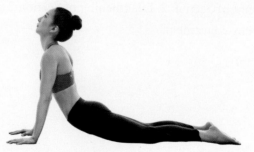

Figure 6.13. *Type P in Upward-facing dog pose (Urdhva Mukha Svanasana).*

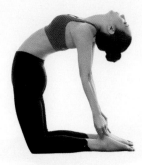

Figure 6.14. *Type P in Camel pose (Ustrasana).*

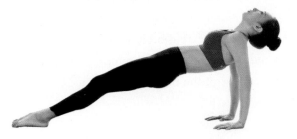

Figure 6.15. *Type P in Upward plank pose (Purvottanasana).*

In backward bends, it is difficult to extend the lumbar spine if the extension commences from the hip joints. A more effective way of preparation is to start with expanding the chest and extending the lumbar area.

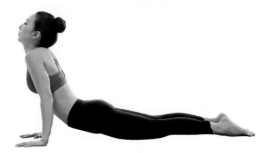

Figure 6.16. *Type P in Upward-facing dog pose (Urdhva Mukha Svanasana) before adjustment.*

In addition, because of the excessive curve of the thoracic vertebrae (kyphosis), it is easy for Type P to elevate the shoulder blades and carry out an internal rotation of the shoulder joints.

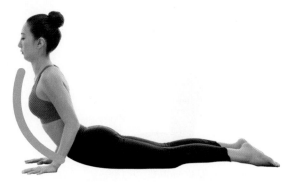

Figure 6.17. *Type P in Cobra pose (Bhujangasana) with adjustment 1.*

As shown in Figure 6.17, lumbar extension is achieved more effectively by lowering the shoulders and expanding the chest in Cobra pose. It is an effective single-section pose for lengthening Section 2 of the front line.

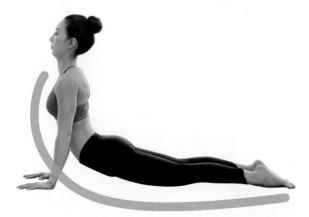

Figure 6.18. *Type P in Upward-facing dog pose (Urdhva Mukha Svanasana) with adjustment 2.*

When Section 2 of the front line is fully lengthened, the Cobra pose can be transformed into the Upward-facing dog pose by lifting the pelvis, thighs, and knees off the ground. In turn, this will lengthen Section 3 of the front line and the pose will be completed, as shown in Figure 6.18.

Locust Pose and Bow Pose

The purpose of these poses is to strengthen Section 2 of the back line (especially the erector spinae muscles), which has become weak and long for Type P.

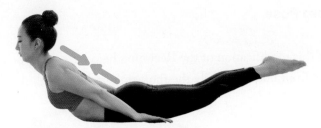

Figure 6.19. *Type P in Locust pose (Salabhasana).*

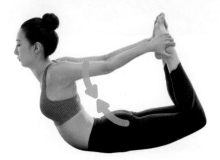

Figure 6.20. *Type P in Bow pose (Dhanurasana).*

Cobra Pose

The purpose of the pose is to lengthen Section 2 of the front line, as an addition to the previously suggested work in Locust and Bow poses.

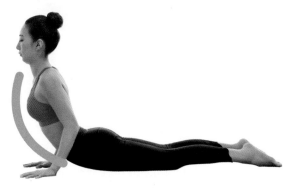

Figure 6.21. *Type P in Cobra pose (Bhujangasana).*

Reclining Hero Pose

The purpose of this modification of the Reclining hero pose for Type P is to lengthen Section 2 of the front line (especially the thoracic vertebrae) with the use of a bolster.

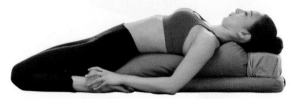

Figure 6.22. *Type P in the modified Reclining hero pose.*

Little Thunderbolt Pose

The purpose of this simple modification of Laghu Vajrasana, shown in Figure 6.23, is to lengthen all the front line of the body (the thoracic vertebrae and lumbar regions) with the help of a yoga wheel.

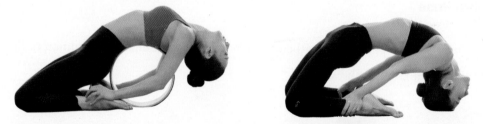

Figure 6.23. *Left: Type P in the Little thunderbolt pose (Laghu Vajrasana). Right: final manifestation of this pose—Type N.*

Pigeon Pose

The purpose of this modification of the Pigeon pose is to lengthen Section 2 of the front line (the thoracic vertebrae and lumbar regions) with the help of a yoga wheel.

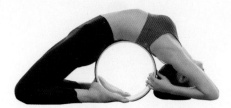 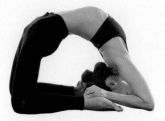

Figure 6.24. *Left: Type P in the modified Pigeon pose (Kapotasana). Right: final manifestation of this pose.*

Type P—Adjustments in Triangle Pose*

Section Imbalances

It is common to observe in Type P that the back line of Section 2 is longer than the front line. The adjustments should focus on creating a balance between the length of Section 2 on both back and front lines.

Imbalances in the Joints

In Triangle pose, the flexed thoracic and lumbar regions and internally rotated shoulders need to be brought back to a neutral position, working in one plane.

---

*My next book about yoga symmetrical imbalances will cover side-bending poses in more detail.

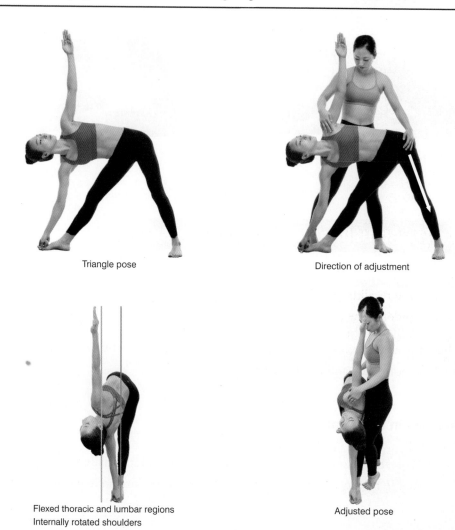

Triangle pose

Direction of adjustment

Flexed thoracic and lumbar regions
Internally rotated shoulders

Adjusted pose

Figure 6.25. *Type P in Triangle pose (Trikonasana) and direction of adjustment back to one plane.*

7

Adjustments for Type A

• • • • • •

The purpose of the adjustments for Type A is to counteract the sectional imbalances.

As you recall from Chapter 3, Type A has an exaggerated anterior pelvic tilt and lumbar lordosis; the hip flexors and erector spinae are strong, whereas the hip extensors and rectus abdominis muscles are weak. This type is also characterized by the outward expansion of energy.

Section 2 of the back line can be lengthened through forward bends, while Section 3 of the front line can be lengthened through backward bends.

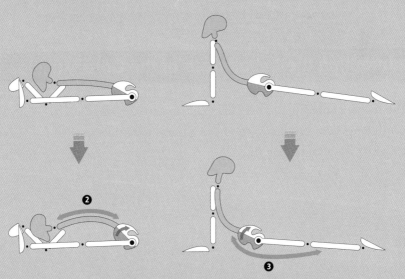

Figure 7.1. *Type A: counteracting the imbalances of the front and back lines.*

Restoring the Direction of the Joint Movements

In Type A, hip extension and lumbar flexion are not fully activated, because of long and weak gluteus maximus and rectus abdominis muscles. Type A should therefore work on strengthening the hip extensor and lumbar flexor.

The left image of Figure 7.2 illustrates the imbalance of Type A; the right image shows the opposite pattern of Type P.

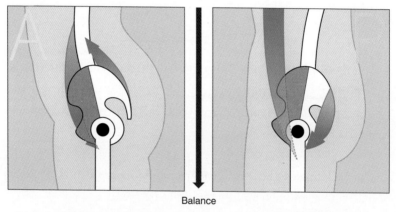

Balance

Figure 7.2. *Type A: Short and strong muscles: psoas and erector spinae (blue). Type P: Short and strong muscles: rectus abdominis and gluteus maximus (blue).*

Counteracting the Imbalances of the Core Muscles

When the rectus abdominis muscle is strengthened, the short erector spinae muscles will lengthen; similarly, when the gluteus maximus muscle is strengthened, the short psoas muscle will lengthen.

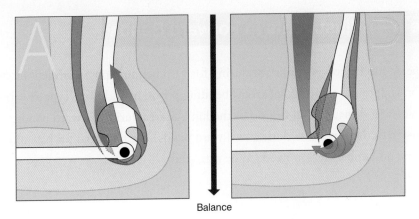

Balance

Figure 7.3.
Type A:
*Blue: **strong** psoas, erector spinae.*
*Red: **weak** rectus abdominis, gluteus maximus.*

Type P:
*Blue: **strong** rectus abdominis, gluteus maximus.*
*Red: **weak** psoas, erector spinae.*

Reversing the Imbalance in Breathing

Induce a balance between inhalation and exhalation by focusing more on the exhalation pattern.

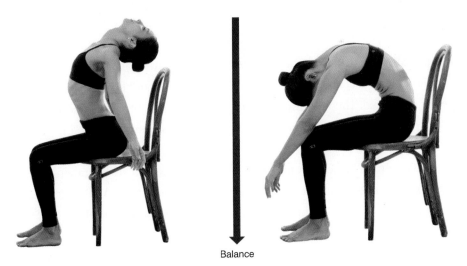

Balance

Figure 7.4. *Inhalation pattern and exhalation pattern.*

Type A—Adjustments in Forward Bends

For Type A, hip flexion is dominant during forward bending poses, while lumbar extension is dominant during backward bending poses. In addition, Type A is prone to experiencing difficulties in flexion of the lumbar area during forward bends and in extension of the hip joints during backward bends. The potential for hip joint extension and lumbar flexion needs to be activated.

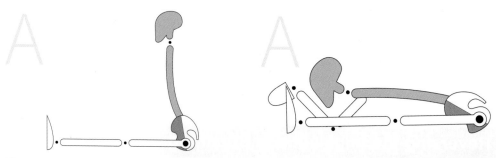

Figure 7.5. *Type A forward bend pattern.*

In forward bending poses, maximizing lumbar flexion while minimizing hip flexion is the most effective prescription for recovering postural and breathing balance for Type A.

When hip flexion is the main habitual/automatic action in a forward bend, a practitioner will not feel any pull or strain, as the iliopsoas and erector spinae muscles are already shortened. The repetition of this pattern will be automatic and may cause even more profound imbalances of anterior pelvic tilt and lordosis.

Instead, while initiating the forward bend, Type A will benefit from drawing the sit bones together and flexing at the lumbar spine; this way, Type A will first create lumbar flexion and then combine it with hip joint flexion more efficiently.

At this point, one may feel the erector spinae and the quadratus lumborum muscles lengthen and the rectus abdominis muscle contract. This is likely to be an unusual sensation for Type A practitioners.

Here is little tip on how to lengthen Section 2 of the back line in a forward bend with straight knees. This may benefit those who struggle despite attempts to curl their tailbone or lengthen their lumbar region.

Initiate a posterior pelvic tilt with the knees bent at first. Then press the heels down, contract the hamstrings, and draw the sit bones together. By doing this, you create posterior pelvic tilt, which enables effective contraction of the rectus abdominis and gluteus maximus muscles. This makes it easier for the lumbar region of Section 2 of the back line to lengthen and flex.

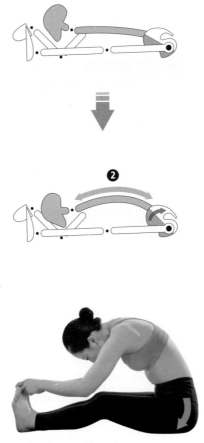

Figure 7.6. *Correction for the Seated forward bend pose.*

When the strength of the abdomen is developed during forward bends, then another common problem for Type A—lifting the buttocks up in Low plank pose—can be resolved. As the abdomen strengthens through the consistent action of drawing it in, movements such as jump backs improve, since the body becomes lighter and less arm power is required. These are the fruits of applying Mula Bandha with posterior pelvic tilt.

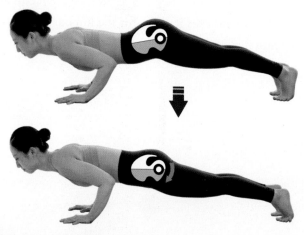

Figure 7.7. *Low plank pose (Chaturanga Dandasana) and the action of Mula Bandha with posterior pelvic tilt.*

Type A—Adjustments in Backward Bends

In most of the multi-section backward bending positions, such as the Upward-facing dog or Camel poses, it is common to find Type A using the hip joints incorrectly and predominantly relying on lumbar extension.

Before initiating backward bends, it is important to prepare the inactive hip joints. If the tailbone is pushed inward and a posterior pelvic tilt is intentionally created, the hip joint will extend first and lumbar extension will follow naturally for Type A.

For those with a severe anterior pelvic tilt and an extremely short psoas, however, it is difficult to awaken the sensation of posterior pelvic tilt, no matter how hard they try to lengthen the hip joints in preparation for the backward bend postures.

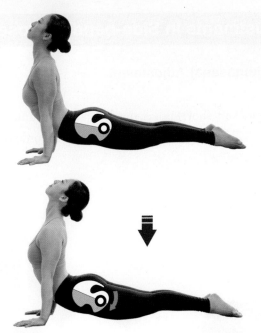

Figure 7.8. *Upward-facing dog pose (Urdhva Mukha Svanasana) correction.*

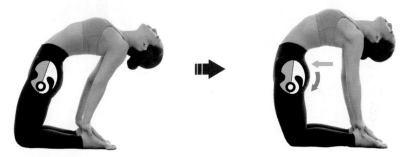

Figure 7.9. *Camel pose (Ustrasana) and adjustment.*

At this point, the rectus abdominis muscles, located between the pubic bones and the sternum, need to be intentionally contracted and guide the lumbar spine into flexion. At the same time, the gluteus maximus muscles and hamstrings will contract and guide the hip joints into extension. Although such a move will hinder the extension of the lumbar joints, it is a step-by-step approach to awakening the sensation of posterior pelvic tilt. It has a surprisingly huge success rate for balancing backward bends in Type A.

With these actions, after extension of the hip joints and contraction of the abdomen, the abdominal muscles can be slowly lengthened while completing the lumbar extension. Such an approach is effective for Type A, as they already have a good sense of lumbar extension.

Type A—Adjustments in Side-bending Poses

Triangle Pose (Trikonasana) Adjustment

Because of the tight (locked-short) psoas, quadratus lumborum, and erector spinae muscles, the buttocks will be pushed outward, resulting in lordosis and excessive extension in the lumbar spine.

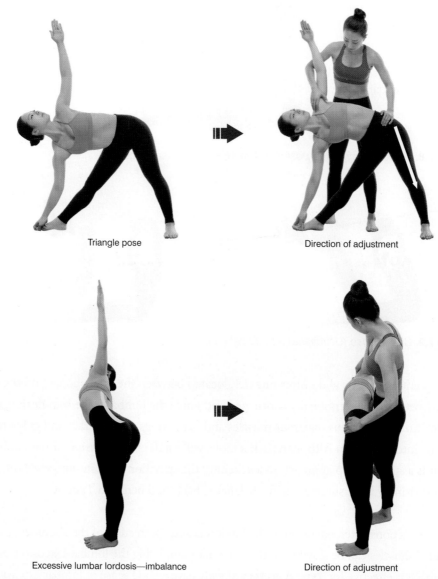

Triangle pose

Direction of adjustment

Excessive lumbar lordosis—imbalance

Direction of adjustment

Figure 7.10. *Type A in Triangle pose (Trikonasana) and direction of adjustment back to one plane.*

Reduce lumbar lordosis by drawing the sit bones together (engage Mula Bandha and gently contract the gluteus muscles) and contracting the abdominal muscles.

Exert strength on the back leg toward the little toe (foot inversion).

Extended Side Angle Pose (Parsvakonasana)

In Parsvakonasana on the right side, to create a solid foundation the adjuster can first use their left leg under the right hip joint of the practitioner. Then, the right hand of the adjuster can support and gently draw the right knee of the practitioner laterally. Finally, the left hand of the adjuster can pull the pelvis laterally and downward to correct the medial rotation of the hip joints and excessive lumbar lordosis.

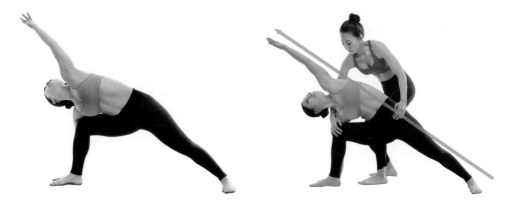

Figure 7.11. *Extended side angle pose (Parsvakonasana)—adjusted.*

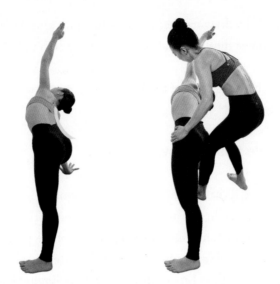

Figure 7.12. *Extended side angle pose (Parsvakonasana), with excessive lumbar lordosis—adjusted.*

Warrior A Pose (Virabhadrasana A)

Because of the anterior pelvic tilt and lumbar lordosis, the psoas and rectus femoris muscles of Type A are typically short and strong. As a result, it is extremely difficult to correct the pelvis to a neutral position in Warrior pose without a help of an adjuster.

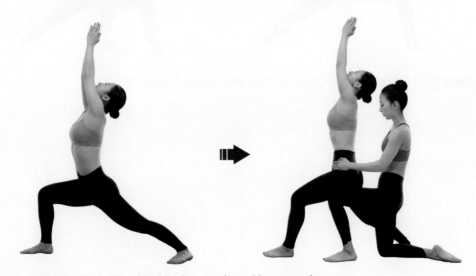

Figure 7.13. *Warrior A pose (Virabhadrasana A) and its correction.*

Using the rectus abdominis muscles and gluteus maximus muscles, the practioner reduces the anterior pelvic tilt by adjusting their pelvis posteriorly. When the muscle imbalance is profound and the proposed above adjustment is not yet helping, the adjuster can assume a low lunge position, facing the same direction as the practitioner; the adjuster places their right knee on the floor and their left knee under the left hip of the practitioner, and draws the pelvis into the neutral position with their hands.

Low Lunge Pose—Lengthening the Psoas

The goal here is to lengthen Section 3 of the front line.

In a low lunge pose, Type A's excessive anterior pelvic tilt can worsen because of their unconscious habits, as seen in the left image of Figure 7.14. This may indirectly strengthen the psoas, which is responsible for hip flexion, and cause it to contract and shorten. To lengthen the psoas, you can push the tailbone in and consciously perform a posterior pelvic tilt.

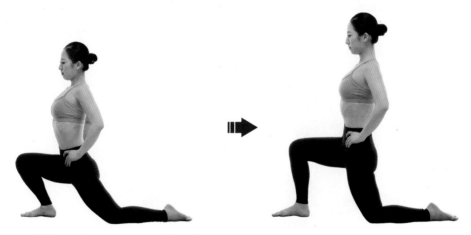

Figure 7.14. *Low lunge pose and its adjustment.*

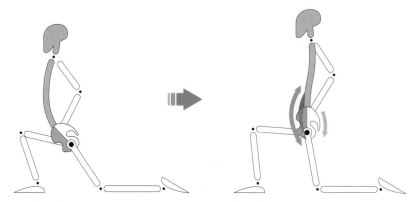

Figure 7.15. *Low lunge pose: graphical representation of the adjustment.*

Reclining Hero Pose—Lengthening the Psoas

The goal here is to lengthen Section 3 of the front line (the psoas).

The adjustment for Reclining hero pose is similar to the adjustment for the Low lunge pose, although the foundation is different. The use of a block under the sacrum is one of the most effective techniques for helping to perform a posterior pelvic tilt.

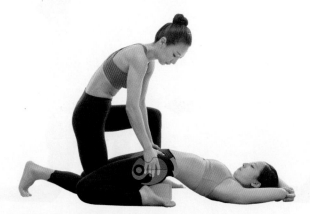

Figure 7.16. *Reclining hero pose (Supta Virasana) adjustment.*

Warrior B Pose (Virabhadrasana B)

Because of relatively weak abductor and gluteus maximus muscles, in Type A the hip joints of the back leg cannot be fully abducted and laterally rotated. As a result, the front leg bears most of the body weight.

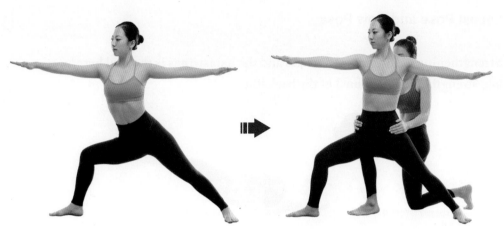

Figure 7.17. *Warrior B pose (Virabhadrasana B) and its adjustment.*

When there is an anterior pelvic tilt condition, due to the short psoas and rectus femoris muscles, it is difficult for the pelvis to maintain a horizontal position and the buttocks tend to protrude outwardly. To balance this posture for Type A, a neutral position of the pelvis should be found by contracting the abdominal and gluteal muscles, and then, on an exhale, the pelvis should be shifted posteriorly, drawing the sit bones together.

Boat Pose—Strengthening the Abdominal Muscles

The intention here is to strengthen Section 2 of the front line.

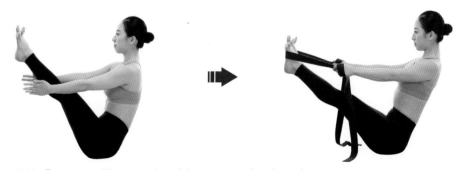

Figure 7.18. *Boat pose (Navasana) and the strap-assisted version.*

Locust Pose and Bow Pose

Strengthening of the gluteal muscles and the hamstrings is the goal here, i.e., strengthening Section 3 of the back line.

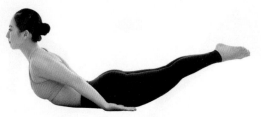

Figure 7.19. *Locust pose (Salabhasana).*

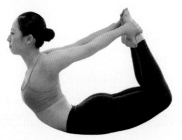

Figure 7.20. *Bow pose (Dhanurasana).*

Upward Plank Pose

For Types A and C, it is common to find that extension happens mostly in the lumbar region and not at the hips (Figure 7.21). By pressing the pointed feet downward and using the gluteal muscles, hip extension can be activated. As there is a tendency for the hip joints to rotate inward, an appropriate adjustment (Figure 7.22) can help to rotate the hips externally, to bring them to a neutral position.

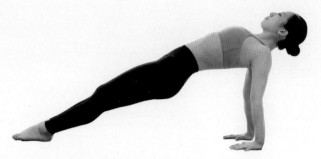

Figure 7.21. *Upward plank pose (Purvottanasana).*

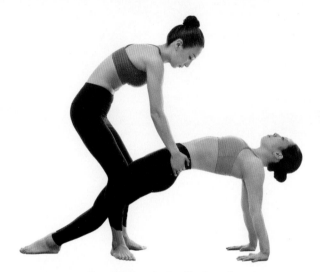

Figure 7.22. *Upward plank pose (Purvottanasana) adjustment.*

8

Adjustments for Type C

Purpose of Adjustments for Type C

Counteracting Sectional Imbalances

Section 2 (lumbar spine area) of the back line can be lengthened through forward bends, while Section 2 (chest area) and Section 3 (pelvic area) of the front line can be lengthened through backward bends.

The primary goal of the adjustment for Type C is to correct excessive anterior pelvic tilt through intentional posterior pelvic tilt.

The secondary goal of adjustment for Type C is to correct excessive thoracic kyphosis through extension of the thoracic vertebrae.

Reversing the Imbalance in Breathing

Induce a balance between inhalation and exhalation by coordinating both inhalation and exhalation patterns (equal inhalations and exhalations).

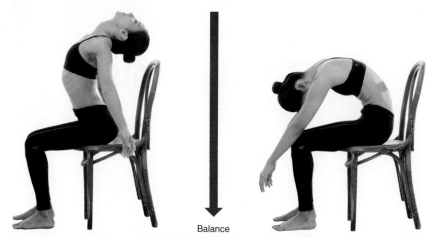

Balance

Figure 8.1. *Inhalation pattern and Exhalation pattern.*

Q7 Why Are There Two Different Goals in the Adjustment for Type C?

Type C is like Type A in terms of the lumbopelvic region, but, at the same time, it is like Type P in terms of the thoracic region (kyphotic-lordotic posture); therefore, it is not easy to categorize this type initially.

In addition, it is difficult to adjust both the lumbopelvic region and the thoracic vertebrae simultaneously, as they require somewhat contradictory actions. Lumbar correction for Type C entails a posterior pelvic tilt, while thoracic correction entails extension of the thoracic vertebrae.

Practitioners will usually have difficulty in performing both lumbar flexion and thoracic extension at the same time. The adjuster may also be confused as to which area to correct first.

In my experience, the initial focus should be on the lumbopelvic region—posterior pelvic tilt and lumbar flexion. Thereafter, the thoracic region gradually needs to be corrected.

If the pelvis and lumbar region recover a neutral balance, the hip joints can establish a stronger foundation; this enables a healthy exchange of energy (prana and apana) downward and upward through the sit bones. When a practitioner restores the balance in the lumbopelvic region, they can focus on lumbar flexion during exhalation and thoracic extension during inhalation, thus combining both goals of the adjustments for Type C.

Adjustment of Thoracic Kyphosis Using a Foam Roller

Using a foam roller under the thoracic area helps to expand the chest region and shoulders of Section 2 of the front line.

In Chapter 6 I suggested that Type P use a yoga wheel for correcting thoracic kyphosis. For Type C, however, I recommend a foam roller, since most of this type's practitioners find the diameter of the wheel too big; a smaller diameter foam roller therefore appears to be a better tool for Type C.

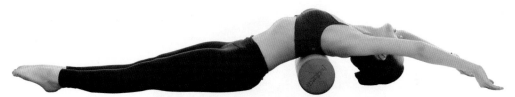

Figure 8.2. *Correcting thoracic kyphosis of Type C with a foam roller.*

Bound Angle Pose B Using a Bolster

The use of a bolster in Baddha Konasana B helps to lengthen the lumbar region of Section 2 of the back line.

As shown in Figure 8.3, pressing down on the bolster with both elbows while exhaling deeply will help to significantly lengthen the lumbar region of Section 2.

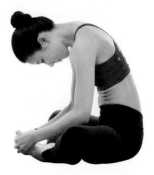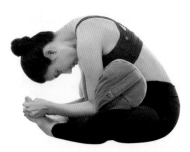

Figure 8.3. *Bound angle pose B (Baddha Konasana B) using a bolster.*

Sleeping Tortoise Pose Using a Bolster

The use of a bolster in Supta Kurmasana helps to lengthen the lumbar region of Section 2 of the back line.

As shown in Figure 8.4, tension can be released in the lumbar spine by raising both legs above the pelvis on a bolster, creating favorable conditions for posterior pelvic tilt.

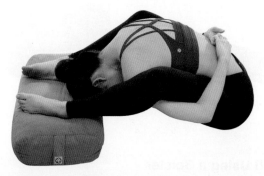

Figure 8.4. *Sleeping tortoise pose (Supta Kurmasana) using a bolster.*

Sage Marichi Pose

In Sage Marichi pose A (Marichyasana A), those with a profound anterior pelvic tilt tend to lift the pelvis on the side of the bent knee too much, leaving most of the body weight on the other side of the body.

The lumbar region of Section 2 of the back line is short in Types A and C, and, because of the limitations in the rotation of the lumbar region, difficulties are often encountered while performing the Sage Marichi pose C (Marichyasana C) as well.

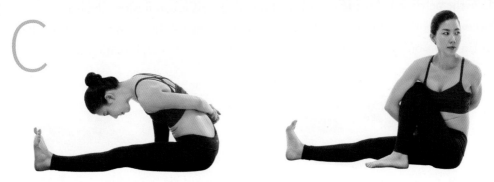

Figure 8.5. *Sage Marichi pose A (Marichyasana A)—Type C. Sage Marichi pose C (Marichyasana C)—Type C.*

The key here is to restore the exhalation pattern in the preparatory stage. On an exhalation, draw the sit bones together, lift the pubic bone, and contract the lower abdomen; these actions will result in a conscious lumbar flexion. Maintaining this lumbar flexion, flex the hips, which will bring about a more balanced forward bend element to Sage Marichi pose A.

While initiating Sage Marichi pose C, exhale deeply, contract the lower abdomen, consciously create a posterior pelvic tilt, and only then enter a rotation. This technique will create more balance between lumbar and hip flexion.

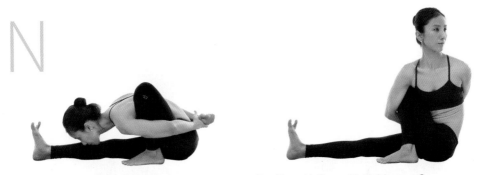

Figure 8.6. *Sage Marichi pose A (Marichyasana A)—Type N. Sage Marichi pose C (Marichyasana C)—Type N.*

Difference Between Bound Angle A and B Poses

Baddha Konasana A is similar to the Seated forward bend pose (Paschimottanasana), where the pelvis is in an anterior tilt and the hip joints are in flexion. The basic objective of both postures is hip flexion, the only difference being in the shape of the legs (in terms of knee flexion and hip joint abduction and lateral rotation).

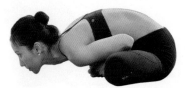 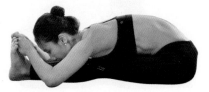

Figure 8.7. *Bound angle pose A (Baddha Konasana A). Seated forward bend pose (Paschimottanasana).*

The Bound angle pose B, on the other hand, is the opposite of the Seated forward bend pose, i.e., the pelvis is in a posterior tilt and the lumbar spine is in flexion. The goal of Baddha Konasana B is to lengthen the lumbar area (erector spinae muscles) of Section 2 of the back line.

If the differences between Bound angle pose A and B are not understood, it is easy to end up focusing only on stretching the adductor muscles in both poses. If the erector spinae muscles in Section 2 of the back line cannot lengthen in Bound angle pose B, the primary purpose of the pose (to establish a strong foundation of the sit bones) will be lost.

Baddha Konasana B, unlike Baddha Konasana A, focuses on lumbar flexion and is a relatively easy posture for Type P, who is used to such forward bending postures.

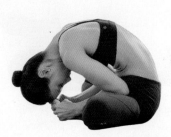 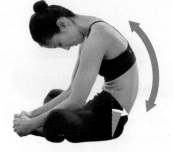

Figure 8.8. *Bound angle pose B (Baddha Konasana B).*

However, it is an extremely difficult pose for Types A and C, who are used to forward bends that focus on hip flexion only. It is not easy for these two types to initiate flexion in Section 2 of the back line, especially the lumbar region, and to create length; therefore, most may find this pose very difficult.

Tortoise/Sleeping Tortoise Pose

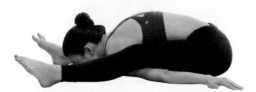 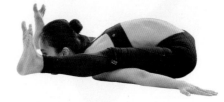

Figure 8.9. *Tortoise pose (Kurmasana).*

People who have trouble performing lumbar flexion will have trouble raising their feet in Kurmasana pose, as depicted in the left image of Figure 8.9. If lumbar flexion is weak, the foundation, which enables drawing the sit bones together, will also be weak.

If Kurmasana pose is performed with force, this could lead to pain in the quadratus lumborum and the erector spinae muscles.

Types A and C will be challenged by Kurmasana, in much the same way they are challenged by Baddha Konasana B, since both poses involve lumbar flexion. With regular practice of both postures, however, they will be able to progress onto the Sleeping tortoise pose.

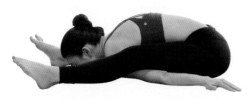 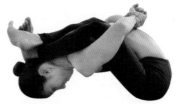

Figure 8.10. *Bound angle pose B (Baddha Konasana). Sleeping tortoise pose (Supta Kurmasana).*

In addition, while the Sage Marichi pose helps to strengthen not only hip joint but also lumbar flexion, both the Boat pose and the Shoulder pressing pose help to strengthen bandha. This is a part of the preparatory process for the Tortoise and Sleeping tortoise poses, which connect the lower body with the rest of the body.

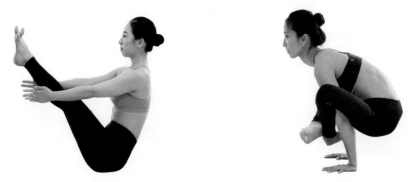

Figure 8.11. *Boat pose (Navasana). Shoulder pressing pose (Bhujapidasana).*

Q8 What Is the Ideal Ratio for Hip and Lumbar Flexion in Forward Bending Poses?

In a seated position, if the practitioner is flexible and can reach a 150-degree forward bend, the hip flexion would be 90 degrees, while the lumbar forward bend would be 60 degrees. This is equivalent to approximately a 3:2 ratio, which is considered appropriate (according to H. David Coulter*; see the table in Figure 8.12). Having said that, opinions vary widely on this matter.

There could be deviations from this ratio, depending on the gender, age group, and flexibility of a person. The value of this ratio also depends on the type of forward bend. For example, whereas a hip to lumbar flexion ratio of 3:2 in the Seated forward bend pose is considered appropriate, this is not the case in the Sage Marichi A pose, where the contribution of hip to lumbar flexion should be balanced more evenly (1:1),

---

*Coulter, H.D. 2017. *Anatomy of Hatha Yoga: A Manual for Students, Teachers, and Practitioners*, Body and Breath, Inc.: Marlboro, VT, USA, p. 278.

because otherwise the symmetric imbalance will worsen. Accordingly, to achieve balance in the Sage Marichy A pose, practitioners need to consciously decrease hip flexion and increase lumbar flexion. The Bound angle B pose is also a representative forward bend pose focusing on lumbar flexion.

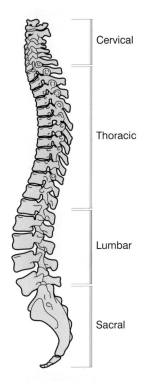

Cervical

Thoracic

Lumbar

Sacral

	T12~L1	L1~L2	L2~L3	L3~L4	L4~L5	L5~S1	T12~S1 total	Hip joint	Spine/hip joint total
Flexion	5	6	8	9	14	18	60	90	150
Extension	4	4	4	9	14	10	45	15	60

Figure 8.12. *This chart estimates the degree of flexion and extension permitted between individual vertebrae between T12 and sacrum in someone who is moderately flexible.*

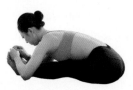 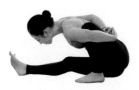 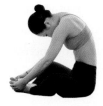

Figure 8.13. *Seated forward bend pose (Paschimottanasana). Sage Marichy A pose (Marichyasana A). Bound angle pose B (Baddha Konasana B).*

For Types A and C, with a severe anterior pelvic tilt, there is a tendency to perform seated forward bends with the prime focus on hip flexion. As it is difficult to flex the lumbar spine in the Sage Marichi pose and bend the lumbar spine completely during the Bound angle pose B, it is almost impossible for these types to bend enough to bring the head close to the feet.

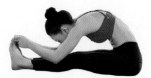 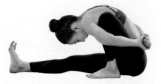 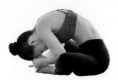

Figure 8.14. *Seated forward bend pose (Paschimottanasana). Sage Marichi pose A (Marichyasana A). Bound angle pose B (Baddha Konasana B).*

The opposite is true for Type P, with a strong posterior pelvic tilt pattern. Type P can enter both Bound angle pose B and Sage Marichi pose A very easily. However, because of the low hip/lumbar flexion ratio in the seated forward bend pose, the back line will be severely bent.

Q9 In the Process of Practicing Yoga We Often Experience Pain. What Are the Basic Principles for Handling Pain?

Pain arises when the body moves away from a state of balance. Pain may also arise as part of the recovery process from an unbalanced to a balanced pattern. In other words, it is important to identify and differentiate the source of pain. Observation is key here.

If the pain is due to an unbalanced posture, it is the body's warning about the unbalanced joint condition. If you distribute the movement of the joints evenly, the pain will disappear.

If we learn to understand the postural type of a practitioner and observe various imbalances in the joints' movements in various postures, we will be able to scan the entire structure of imbalances.

At this point, the basic correction will start with restoring the disrupted lumbopelvic rhythm. When the lumbopelvic rhythm is disrupted, the upper spine will have trouble in its axial extension, while the lower body will form a weak foundation.

When inactive hip joint and lumbar movement directions are awakened, and joint movements in both directions are activated and stability is restored, the lumbopelvic rhythm will return to its natural balance as well.

If both the hip joint and the lumbar spine start moving together in a combined corrective motion, the imbalances of the muscles and all unnecessary stress and energy wastage will disappear. Reconciling with the ground, energy will flow through the spine and guide the pelvis and spine toward restoring balance.

9

Alignment of the Limbs

• • • • • •

S
o far, we have looked mainly at the various imbalances in the spine and pelvic
areas (Sections 2 and 3), and the different correction principles and methods for
the various body types. We should acknowledge, however, that there are limits to
restoring proper function by only correcting the spine and pelvic imbalances.

For the pelvis (Section 3) to return to its neutral position, alignment of the lower body
in Section 4 is required. This is because the energy can only flow through the aligned
legs up to the pelvis and spine when the foundation is fully formed through the solid
connection of the feet with the ground. In addition, to restore balance in the thoracic
vertebrae (Section 2), it is necessary to establish balance in the shoulder blades through
the alignment of the upper limbs.

The traditional Ashtanga Vinyasa Yoga sequence starts with Sun salutations (Surya
Namaskara), which include the Upward-facing dog and Downward-facing dog
poses. Both asanas use all four limbs to form a stable foundation. This incorporation
of traditional poses is not simply for warming up the body. The primary intention of
the beginning sequence is to return to the foundation through the use of these four
limbs poses.

Thereafter, it is essential to establish the lower body foundation from the standing
sequence and guide the pelvis and the spine into balance progressively during the
sitting sequence that follows.

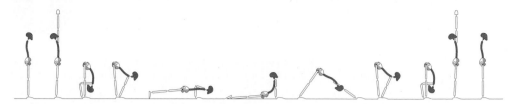

Figure 9.1. *Sun salutation sequence A (Surya Namaskara A).*

Sun Salutation Sequence (Surya Namaskara)

Why Does the Sequence Revolve Around the Dog Pose?

The Downward-facing dog pose in the Sun salutation sequence can be considered a main pose; this is because, while the other poses require only one inhalation or one exhalation each, this pose requires five inhalations and five exhalations.

As well as forming part of the Surya Namaskara sequences in Ashtanga Vinyasa Yoga, the dog poses are used in vinyasa transitions to other postures, and are repeated more than 30 times throughout the practice.

So, why do we start our practice with the dog pose and why did ancient yogis place so much emphasis on these poses?

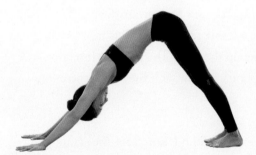

Figure 9.2. *Downward-facing dog pose (Adho Mukha Svanasana).*

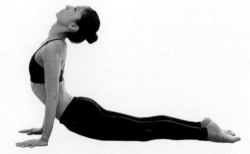

Figure 9.3. *Upward-facing dog pose (Urdhva Mukha Svanasana).*

A Reunion with the Ground Through the Four Limbs

To understand the importance of the dog poses, let us compare them with some of the other poses, e.g., the Cobra pose and the Cat pose.

In the Cobra pose, the lifting of the upper body is mainly achieved by the strength of the spine rather than the use of the hands, which only press lightly against the ground to form the foundation.

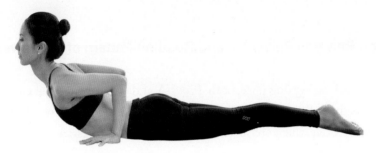

Figure 9.4. *Cobra pose (Bhujangasana).*

In the Cat pose, there are six foundations—hands, knees, and feet—but the transfer of earth energy from the legs to the spine is not as strong as, for example, in the Downward-facing dog pose.

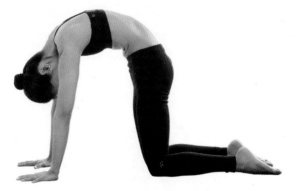

Figure 9.5. *Cat pose (Marjaryasana).*

Unlike the above two asanas, the two dog poses can effectively transfer energy from the earth to the pelvis and spine areas, through the foundations of both the hands and the feet, which are connected to the ground. As mentioned earlier, these are ideal postures for correction purposes. The imbalances in Sections 2 and 3 of the body can be corrected, using the strong energy that is transferred through the four pillars formed by the arms and legs.

We can appreciate the wisdom of the ancient yogis, who developed the four-limbed poses to correct the imbalances which occurred during the evolutionary process from quadruped to biped.

Connection Between Pelvic Tilt and Rotation Pattern of the Lower Limbs

In the Downward-facing dog pose, both Types A and C have an imbalance, where Section 2 of the back line is short, while Section 3 is long. In other words, from a joint movement perspective, there are severe imbalances due to excessive lumbar lordosis and anterior pelvic tilt.

Type P, on the other hand, has an imbalance pattern where Section 2 of the back line is long and Section 3 is short, which indicates imbalances in lumbar flexion and posterior pelvic tilt.

It is common to find a relationship between the lumbopelvic imbalances of Types A and C, and an internal rotation of the lower limbs. In contrast, for Type P there is a connection between their lumbopelvic imbalance and an external rotation of the lower limbs.

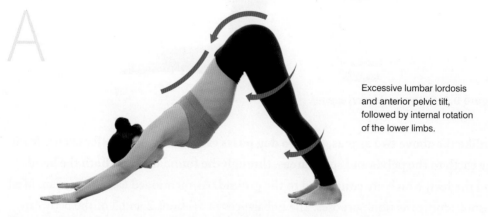

Excessive lumbar lordosis and anterior pelvic tilt, followed by internal rotation of the lower limbs.

Figure 9.6. *Type A in Downward-facing dog pose (Adho Mukha Svanasana).*

P

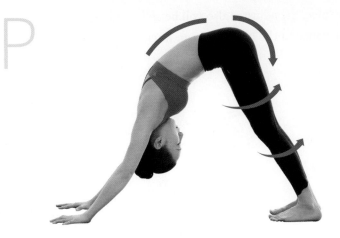

Excessive thoracic kyphosis and posterior pelvic tilt, followed by external rotation of the lower limbs.

Figure 9.7. *Type P in Downward-facing dog pose (Adho Mukha Svanasana).*

How to Observe Imbalances in the Rotation of the Hip Joint

The typical gazing point (drishti) for the Downward-facing dog pose is the belly button. In the case of Types A and C, it is difficult to focus on the belly button because of the excessive anterior pelvic tilt and lumbar lordosis.

One can identify any imbalances in the internal and external rotation of the hip joints by observing the distance between the kneecap and the center line.

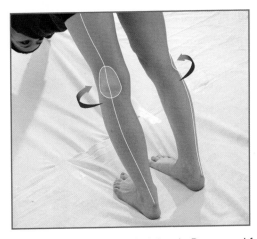

Figure 9.8. *Exaggerated internal rotation of the hip joints in Downward-facing dog pose, identifiable by the position of the knees.*

By observing the back of the knee, the adjuster also will be able to identify and differentiate whether the imbalance in the hip joint is an internal rotation or an external rotation.

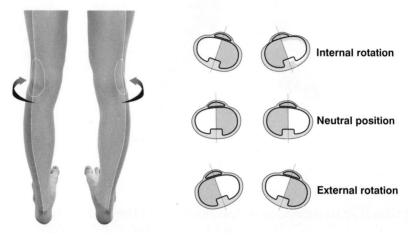

Figure 9.9. *Unbalanced internal rotation of the hip joint.*

Differences Between Rotation of the Hip Joints and the Knee Joints

If the knees come closer to the center line, one could deduce that this arises from internal rotation of the hip joints. Note, this is not due to internal rotation of the knee joints.

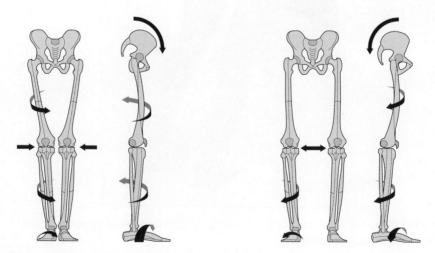

Figure 9.10. *Rotation of the hip joint and the knee joint.*

If the knees are in a straightened position, the hip joints and the knee joints rotate together as one unit. What appears to be an internal rotation of the knee joint is actually caused by the internal rotation of the hip joints.

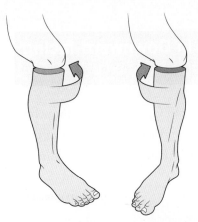

Internal and external rotation of the knee is possible when the knee is bent to an angle of more than 15 degrees. In this situation, if the hip joint remains stationary, the knee joint may move.

Figure 9.11. *Knee rotation with the knee bent to an angle of more than 15 degrees.*

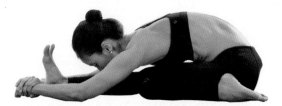

Figure 9.12. *Three-limbed forward bend (Triang Mukha Eka Pada Paschimottanasana).*

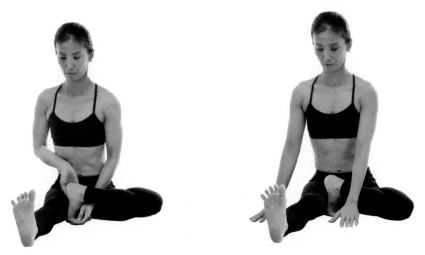

Figure 9.13. *Head to knee forward bend (Janu Sirsasana) C pose preparation.*

There are many seated yoga poses that practice internal and external rotation of the knee joints. The subtle internal and external rotation of the knee joints is essential for stability in meditation poses, such as the Lotus pose.

Correction of the Lower Limbs in Downward-facing Dog Pose

There is a tendency for the hip joints of Types A and C, with an anterior pelvic tilt imbalance condition, to develop an internal rotation pattern. As a result of the internal rotation of the hip joints, there is often an internal rotation of the knee joints and a pronated pattern of the feet.

Type P, with a posterior pelvic tilt condition, has a tendency to exhibit external rotation of the hip joints. Because of the external rotation of the hip joints, there will also tend to be an external rotation of the knee joints and a supinated pattern of the feet.

As imbalances in the lumbar region and pelvis are connected to imbalances of the lower limbs, the correction of lower limb imbalances will also help to correct lumbopelvic imbalances. Moreover, as the hip joints, knees, and feet are connected and work synchronously, any correction made to one of these joints will also lead to correction in the other two joints.

If we look at the overall relationship between the feet, knees, hip joints, pelvis, and lumbar spine and consider them as a whole, an effective correction is possible.

Corrective Method for the Knees

First of all, the common condition whereby the knees seem to rotate internally for Types A and C is usually connected to the hyperextension condition of the knees. Therefore, by bending the overextended knees slightly and moving the inner-facing kneecaps toward the neutral position, it is possible to correct the internal rotation of the hip joints and the pronation of the feet.

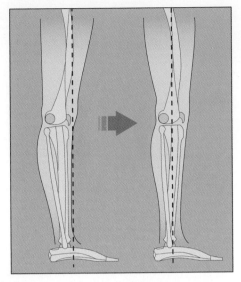

When the knee joints turn toward the center line on the left, the overextension condition of the knees can be identified.

Figure 9.14. *Knee correction technique for Types A and C.*

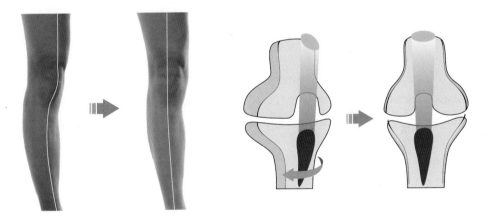

Figure 9.15. *Types A and C correction: internal rotation, hyperextended knee → correction of the knee to a neutral position with balanced extension.*

In the case of Type P, the external rotation of the hip joint and supination of feet can be corrected by engaging the slightly flexed knee in a balanced extension and adjusting the outward-facing kneecap toward the neutral position by moving the knees.

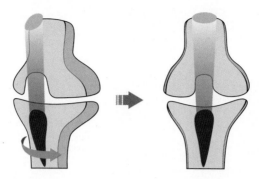

Figure 9.16. *Type P correction of the knee to a neutral position with balanced extension— externally rotated knee.*

Adjustment for the Feet

Pressing the Roots of the Toes

As shown in Figure 9.17, the heel of the foot is lifted up by dorsiflexion. The metatarsophalangeal joints (MTP) are also bent (extended), which is performed by the metatarsal bones and proximal bones of the toes. These are some of the most important joints among those that help to form a stable foundation between the feet and the ground. We could call these the *roots* of the toes. The roots of the toes are evenly distributed when executing the Downward-facing dog pose or when standing upright, and this is extremely important in building up the foundation of the feet.

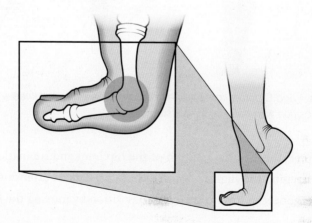

Figure 9.17. *Toes and their roots.*

Figure 9.18 shows the three types of arch in the foot:

1. From the root of the big toe (A) to the heel of the foot (C), which forms an *inner longitudinal arch* connecting both joints.
2. From the root of the little toe (B) to the heel of the foot (C), which forms an *outer longitudinal arch*.

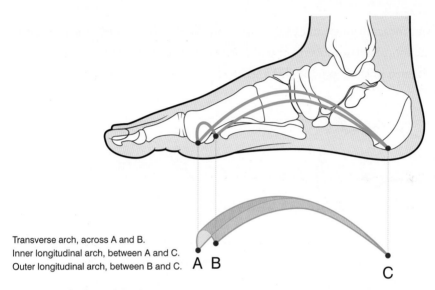

Transverse arch, across A and B.
Inner longitudinal arch, between A and C.
Outer longitudinal arch, between B and C.

Figure 9.18. *Arches of the foot.*

3. In between the root of the big toe (A) and the root of the little toe (B), which forms a *transverse arch* across the width of the foot.

When the roots of both the big toe and the little toe are pressed down evenly in a balanced manner, the transverse and longitudinal arches will also be formed in a balanced manner.

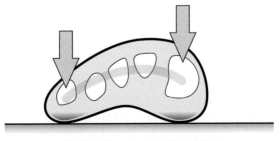

Create balance in strength by pressing down using the big toe and little toe.

Figure 9.19. *Balancing the foot.*

Correcting Pronation and Supination Imbalances of the Feet

Because of the tendency for the hip joints to rotate internally, Types A and C are prone to overexerting pressure on the root of the big toe. Consequently, as the transverse arch and external longitudinal arch collapse, pronation (eversion) imbalances in the feet can be observed.

As a corrective measure, one can exert pressure on the root of the little toe to restore balance to the foot. Such a movement will not only benefit the foot, but also help in recovering balance in the hip joint and knees.

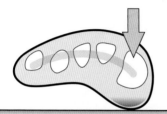   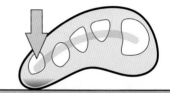

Pronation (eversion) imbalance occurs when the strength at the little toe is weak.   Supination (inversion) imbalance occurs when the strength at the big toe is weak.

Figure 9.20. *Pronation imbalance.*   **Figure 9.21.** *Supination imbalance.*

Type P, on the other hand, is prone to overexerting pressure on the root of the little toe, because of the tendency for the hip joints to rotate externally. Consequently, as the transverse arch and inner longitudinal arch collapse, supination (inversion) imbalances of feet can be observed.

As a corrective measure, one can exert pressure on the root of the big toe to restore balance to the foot. Such a movement is useful in regaining balance in the hip joint and knees.

Adjustments for the Hip Joints

Types A and C have a tendency to internally rotate the hip joints. By holding Section 3 on the front line (the quadriceps) and pulling back, the adjuster can rotate the hip joints outward and correct to a neutral position.

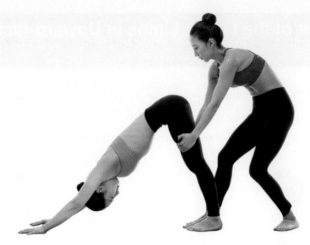

Figure 9.22. *Correction of the internal rotation of the hip joints for Type A in Downward-facing dog pose.*

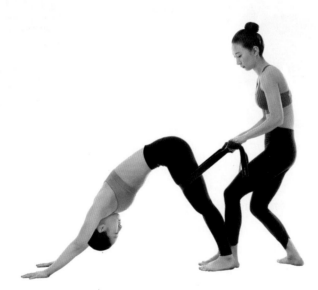

Figure 9.23. *Correction of the internal rotation of the hip joints using a strap or belt for Type A in Downward-facing dog pose.*

As Type P has a tendency to rotate the hips externally, however, the outward rotation will be intensified if both legs are pulled more laterally backward. Therefore, if the adjuster crosses their arms in an X shape and pulls the thighs medially backward, this will help to rotate the hip joints internally into a neutral position.

Adjustment of the Lower Limbs in Upward-facing Dog Pose

Types A and C, with their anterior pelvic tilt condition, have a tendency to internally rotate the hip joints when executing the Upward-facing dog pose. As a result, a pronation (eversion) pattern of the feet can be observed.

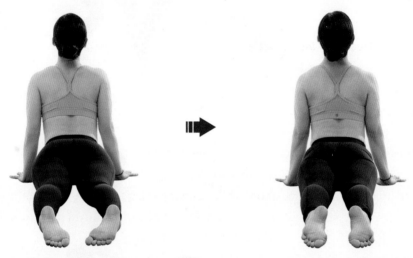

Figure 9.24. *Types A and C in Upward-facing dog pose (Urdhva Mukha Svanasana) and the correction of the feet.*

As illustrated in the left image of Figure 9.24, when the Upward-facing dog pose is executed by Types A and C, it is common to observe imbalances in the shape of the foundation, where the big toes are located near to each other, while the heels of the feet are far away from each other, forming an unbalanced shape.

Similarly, the unbalanced shape of the feet reflected in the left diagram of Figure 9.25 shows the weakened root of the little toe tilting upward; this is because of the pronation (eversion) foot pattern.

When lying in a prone position on the ground, only the top of the little toe is pressed against the ground (as shown in the right image of Figure 9.24). As a result, only the little-toe side on the dorsum of the foot becomes the foundation, and a typical imbalance in the foot shape is developed in Types A and C.

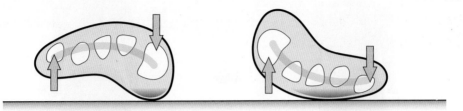

Figure 9.25. *Direction of the top of the little toe pressing against the ground.*

This imbalance characterized by pronation of foot is a condition that is common among children who sit frequently in a particular position (e.g., kneeling or Virasana).

As it is easy for the direction of the feet to go haywire in prone positions (e.g., Upward dog or Cobra), it is important for the teacher to hold the heels of the feet in place to rotate them into a neutral position, while allowing the practitioner to feel the corrected position. It is also beneficial for a practitioner to observe their own posture and make the necessary adjustments.

When executing the Upward-facing dog pose, Type P, with a posterior pelvic tilt condition, tends to rotate the hip joints externally; this can be observed by a supination pattern of the feet. The left image of Figure 9.26 shows that, when Type P executes the Upward-facing dog pose, the heels of the feet are close to each other, while the big toes are far apart from each other. This is a commonly observed imbalance in the shape of the feet for Type P.

As seen in the left image of Figure 9.27, the root of the big toe in this position is weak and therefore tends to lift upward, resulting in imbalance. In the prone position, as shown in the right image of the same figure, only the side of the big toe touches the ground. As a result, typical imbalances in the foot shape are developed.

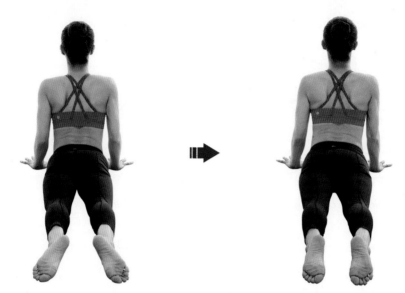

Figure 9.26. *Type P in Upward-facing dog pose (Urdhva Mukha Svanasana) and the correction of the feet.*

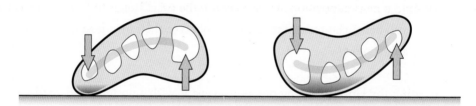

Figure 9.27. *Direction of the top of the big toe pressing against the ground.*

Common Imbalance of the Foot in Types A and C: Pronation (Eversion)

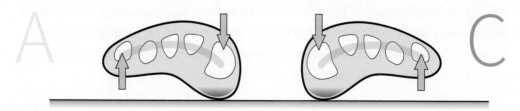

Figure 9.28. *Sole of foot foundation in standing pose for Types A and C.*

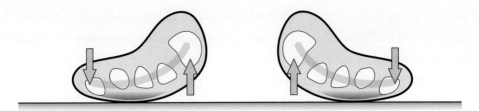

Figure 9.29. *Dorsum of foot foundation in Upward-facing dog pose for Types A and C.*

Common Imbalance of the Foot in Type P: Supination (Inversion)

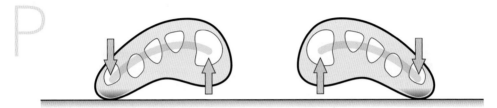

Figure 9.30. *Sole of foot foundation in standing pose for Type P.*

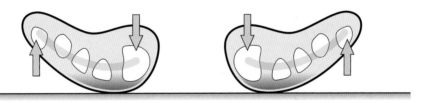

Figure 9.31. *Dorsum of foot foundation in Upward-facing dog pose for Type P.*

Q10 Should the Gluteus Maximus Be in a Contracted State or Relaxed State When Executing the Upward-facing Dog Pose?

The answer to this depends on the type of imbalance in pelvic tilt and the type of rotation pattern of the hip joint.

When executing multi-section backward bends, such as Upward-facing dog pose, Types A and C are more prone to lumbar extension than hip joint extension, because of their anterior pelvic tilt condition. It is common to observe that the gluteal muscles are completely relaxed and the feet are extremely pronated. In such cases, because of the severity of the unbalanced internal rotation of the hip joints, it is necessary to actively contract the gluteus maximus in order to extend the hip joints, and to strengthen the external rotation movements of these joints in order to restore a neutral position.

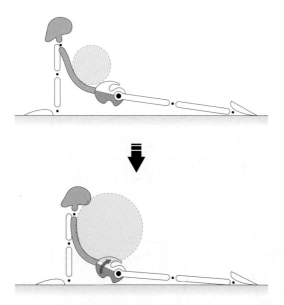

Through conscious effort to correct the posterior pelvic tilt, by extending just the lumbar joints and creating a small circle on an unbalanced backward bend curve, one can extend the lumbar and hip joints together and make a big circle on a balanced backward bend curve.

Figure 9.32. *Adjustment for Type P in the Upward-facing dog pose.*

Because of the posterior pelvic tilt condition, Type P has difficulty in extending their lumbar spine sufficiently, but not their hip joints. It is common to find the gluteal muscles excessively contracted and the feet supinated. With such severe external rotation of the hip joints, it is beneficial for Type P to extend the lumbar area by relaxing the gluteal muscles, thus consciously restoring a neutral position.

Such issues of contracting or relaxing the gluteal muscles, depending on the body type and observations, will constantly surface, and the solution will be applicable not only to the Upward-facing dog pose but also to other multi-section backward bends, such as the Camel pose.

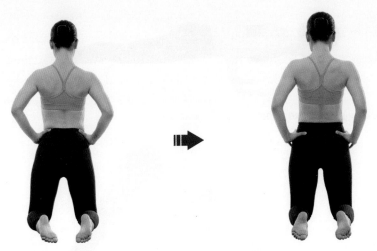

Figure 9.33. *Type A in Camel pose (Ustrasana) and the correction.*

Q11 We Discussed the Relationship Between Lumbopelvic Area and Lower Limbs. Now, What About the Upper Limbs? What Are the Important Arm Balance Poses in Developing Stability of the Upper Body?

There are many poses or elements of asana which require long-term practice to achieve, such as the jump through in vinyasa and the handstand pose. It is common to see many practitioners attempting to accomplish these poses in one go and sustaining injuries or experiencing pain as a result. It is important to always keep the purpose and goal in mind. The purpose of arm balance poses is to restore balance between the lower body and the upper body, by restoring stability to the upper limbs.

The Sun salutation sequence of vinyasa down and vinyasa up (Downward-facing and Upward-facing dog poses, as well as some of the other poses in the sequence) is ideal for developing the stability of the upper body through the practice of the four-limbed foundation poses.

In particular, vinyasa 4 of the Sun salutation—Low plank (Chaturanga Dandasana)—and vinyasa 6—Downward-facing dog (Adho Mukha Svanasana)—are the most important basic poses which, through regular practice, will help the body to restore its neutral position and stability of the upper limbs. Through these poses, the stable equilibrium of the shoulders and shoulder blades can be restored.

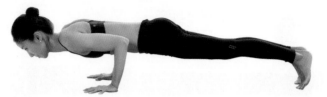

Figure 9.34. *Low plank pose (Chaturanga Dandasana).*

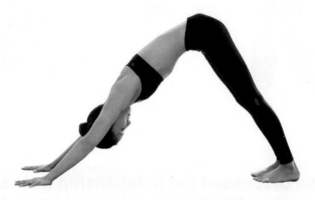

Figure 9.35. *Downward-facing dog pose (Adho Mukha Svanasana).*

Apart from these, poses such as the Shoulder pressing pose, Firefly pose, Crow pose, and Handstand pose are important for attaining vertical balance. To restore the balance in the spinal pelvic areas and limbs, which form the core of the human body, continuous practice over a long period of time is required.

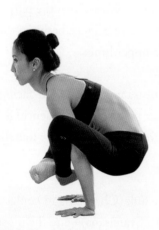

Figure 9.36. *Shoulder pressing pose (Bhujapidasana).*

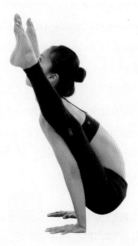

Figure 9.37. *Firefly pose (Tittibhasana).*

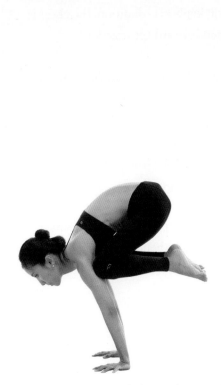

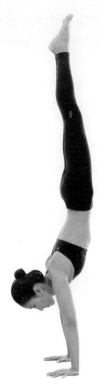

Figure 9.38. *Crow pose (Bakasana).*

Figure 9.39. *Handstand pose (Adho Mukha Vrksasana).*

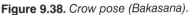
Imbalances in the Shoulder Blades and Shoulder Joints

If the shoulder blades are not able to maintain balance while standing upright, and habitually tilt forward (protraction) or arch backward (retraction), this unbalanced posture pattern could become permanent. Rather than attributable to imbalances in the shoulder blade itself, it is more likely to be due to the compensation effect that arises from imbalances in the pelvis and spine.

In the case of Type A, with anterior pelvic tilt and lumbar lordosis condition, the chest is pushed outward, while the shoulder blades are pushed backward (retraction). (See the Mountain pose in the Appendix for a visual reference.)

For Type P, with posterior pelvic tilt and thoracic kyphosis condition, the chest is curved inward and the shoulder blades are pushed forward (protraction).

For Type C, with anterior pelvic tilt and thoracic kyphosis condition, the chest is curved inward and the shoulder blades are pushed forward (protraction).

One interesting point for Type A is that not only are the shoulder blades retracted, but also the shoulder joints are rolled outward, thus resulting in the palms facing outward when the arms are straightened in an upright standing position.

On the other hand, since the shoulder blades of both Type P and Type C are protracted, the shoulder joints are also rotated internally, hence resulting in the backs of the hands facing outward.

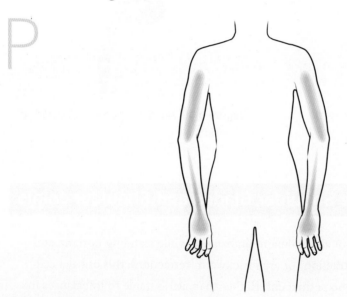

Figure 9.40. *Type P imbalance of the upper limbs: protraction of the shoulder blades and internal rotation of the shoulder joints.*

Adjustment of the Upper Limbs in the Downward-facing Dog Pose

Common imbalances observed in the Downward-facing dog pose executed by Type A are retraction of the shoulder blades and internal rotation of the shoulder joints.

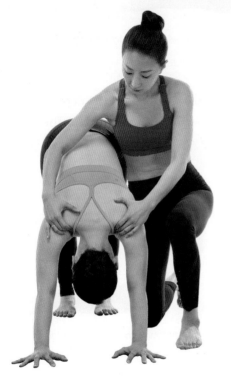

Note: The reason why imbalances in internal rotation of the shoulder joints commonly occur in the Downward-facing dog pose as compared with the Upright standing pose (imbalances in external rotation of the shoulder joints) is that, because of the anterior pelvic tilt and lumbar lordosis condition of Type A, internal rotation of the lower body occurs, leading to a weakened lower body foundation. In consequence, the weight of the body falls mostly on the upper body and the arms. The shoulder joints are therefore excessively internally rotated in an attempt to compensate for the body weight.

As a result, the foundations of both the upper body and the lower body develop internal rotation imbalances.

Figure 9.41. *Adjustment of the upper limbs in the Downward-facing dog pose.*

The direction of the correction should be to widen the distance between the shoulder blades (protraction), and to rotate the shoulder joints laterally toward a neutral position.

Common imbalances observed in the Upward-facing dog pose executed by Type P and Type C are elevation and protraction of the shoulder blades and internal rotation of the shoulder joints.

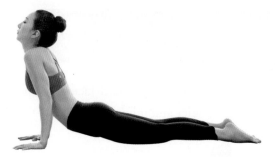

Figure 9.42. *Type P imbalance in Upward-facing dog pose: elevated and protracted shoulder blades, and internal rotation of the shoulder joints.*

The direction of the correction should be to lower the shoulder blades (depression) and push them backward (retraction), and to rotate the shoulder joints laterally toward a neutral position.

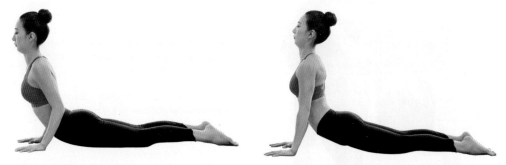

Figure 9.43. *Correction of Type P in Upward-facing dog pose: lower the shoulder blades and push backward, and rotate the shoulder joints laterally.*

The cause of such imbalances is the unbalanced patterns of the lumbar spine and pelvis, which result in a compensation effect on limb movements. Having said that, there is a limit to the correction of the imbalances in the limbs themselves. It is therefore necessary to practice the corrections for the lumbar spine, pelvis, and lower body, presented in Chapters 5 to 8, as an integral process in order to achieve the fundamental effects of the correction.

Specific Goals for the Upper Limbs

Imbalances in the postures usually originate from the pelvis and spread not only to the hip joint and lower body, but also to the thoracic vertebrae and shoulder blades of the upper limbs through a series of joint movement patterns. Upper limb movements in yoga asanas are designed to counter such imbalances in the shoulder blades and upper limbs.

Corrective Limb Poses for Type A

Eagle Pose: Protraction of Scapulae and Internal Rotation of Shoulder Joints

The upper body movements in Garudasana are designed to correct the retraction of the shoulder blades and external rotation of the shoulder joints in Type A. As shown in Figure 9.44, the upper body movements comprise moving the shoulder blades forward. The rotation of the shoulder joints differs, however, between the bottom left arm and the top right arm: the image shows that the shoulder joint of the bottom left arm is rotating internally, whereas the shoulder joint of the top right arm is rotating externally. Repeat the pose with the left arm on top of the right arm; the rotation of the shoulder joints will change accordingly.

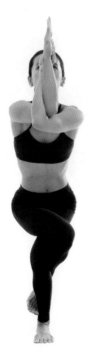
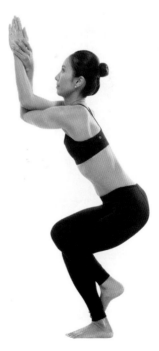

Figure 9.44. *Eagle pose (Garudasana).*

Intense Side Stretch Pose: Inward Rotation of Shoulder Joints

Although this is a posture which moves the shoulder blades into retraction, and might therefore not seem to be applicable to Type A, the action of joining the palms behind the back (Anjali Mudra) is difficult for many Type A practitioners; the reason for this is Type A's limited inward rotation of the shoulder joints. Thus, it is an appropriate pose for the correction of Type A shoulder imbalance. If it is not possible to execute Anjali Mudra, it is recommended to start with an easier internal rotation pose by holding onto both elbows.

Corrective Limb Poses for Type P and Type C

A perfect correction for counteracting the protraction of the shoulder blades and internal rotation of the shoulder joints in Types P and C is to execute Wide-legged forward bend C, Bow, and Camel poses, which promote shoulder blade retraction and external rotation of the shoulder joints.

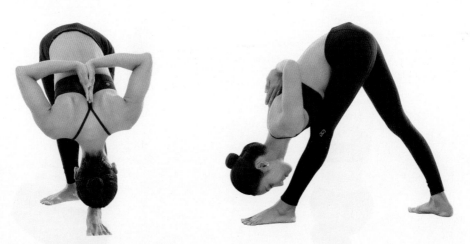

Figure 9.45. *Intense side stretch pose (Parsvottanasana).*

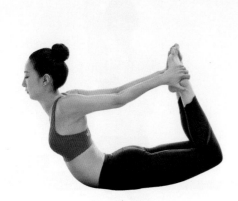

Figure 9.46. *Bow pose (Dhanurasana).*

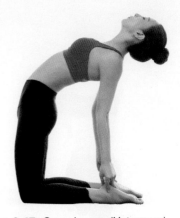

Figure 9.47. *Camel pose (Ustrasana).*

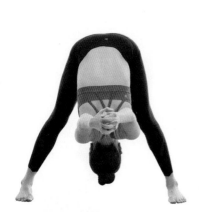
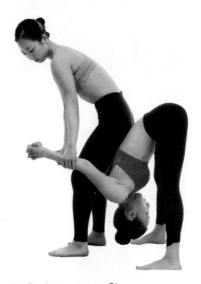

Figure 9.48. *Wide-legged forward bend pose C (Prasarita Padottanasana C).*

The Cow face pose counteracts retraction of the shoulder blades and internal/external rotation of the left and right arms.

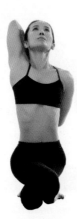
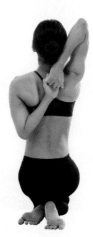

Figure 9.49. *Cow face pose (Gomukhasana): retraction of the shoulder blades, internal rotation of the bottom arm, and external rotation of the top arm.*

Eagle Pose: Protraction of Shoulder Blades

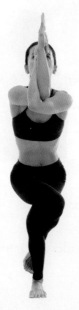
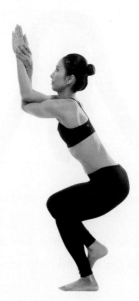

Figure 9.50. *Eagle pose (Garudasana): protraction of the shoulder blades, internal rotation of the bottom arm, and external rotation of the top arm.*

10

Breathing Practices for Postural Balance

• • • • • •

One of the greatest hindrances to attaining postural balance is the sectional imbalances we have discussed so far. The specific adjustments to address the section imbalances are extremely effective at restoring neutrality in the practitioner.

When practicing the "balancing" poses discussed in Chapters 1 to 9, however, you can expect more positive results if these postures are combined with conscious breathing.

Traditionally, the techniques discussed in this chapter were developed by yogis for the effective union of the postures and breathing.

In Chapter 4 we discussed how to create harmony between spinal pelvic movements and breathing, restoring neutrality in the practitioner.

Breathing Mechanisms for Different Body Types

As discussed in Chapter 4, there is a connection between unbalanced posture types and unbalanced breathing patterns. The inhalation pattern is more dominant in Type A, whereas the exhalation pattern is more dominant in Type P.

Because of a lengthened Section 2 on the front line and a shortened Section 2 on the back line, Type A is prone to breathing mechanisms that focus on *thoracic* breathing. For Type A it is easy to expand the chest using the intercostal muscles, but they suffer from weak abdominal muscles.

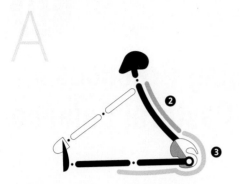
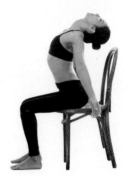

Figure 10.1. *Type A breathing pattern.*

Because of a shortened Section 2 on the front line and a lengthened Section 2 on the back line, Type P is prone to breathing mechanisms that focus on *abdominal* **breathing.** Although they have difficulty expanding the chest using the intercostal muscles, they excel at exhalation using the abdominal muscles.

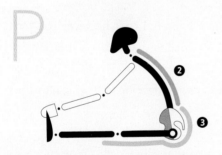
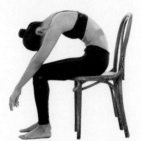

Figure 10.2. *Type P breathing pattern.*

Thoracic Breathing and Abdominal Breathing

Recovering Breathing Imbalances

The torso of the human body is made up of the *thoracic cavity* and the *abdominopelvic cavity*. The pressure within these cavities can be regulated by movement of the muscles of respiration.

Inhalation draws air into the chest area when the pressure within the thoracic cavity is reduced as a result of the expansion of the thorax. The thorax is expanded using the intercostal muscles and diaphragm.

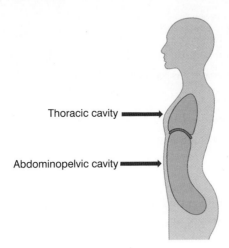

Thoracic cavity

Abdominopelvic cavity

Figure 10.3. *Cavities of the human torso.*

The contraction of the intercostal muscles raises the ribs upward and outward, thus expanding the thoracic cavity. When the diaphragm contracts, its center moves downward and expands the thoracic cavity.

As Section 2 on the front line is long for Type A, while Section 2 on the back line is short, it is easy for them to breathe using the intercostal muscles. In addition, because of the anterior pelvic tilt pattern, downward movement of the diaphragm is not easy.

The breathing mechanism of inhalation using the intercostal muscles with horizontal expansion of the thoracic cavity is known as *thoracic breathing*.

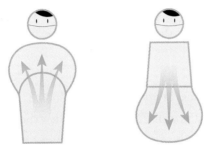

Figure 10.4. *Patterns of thoracic and abdominal breathing.*

On the other hand, it is not easy for Type P to inhale using the intercostal muscles because of a short Section 2 on the front line and a long Section 2 on the back line. On the contrary, the posterior pelvic tilt condition makes downward movement of the diaphragm easier.

The breathing mechanism of inhalation that uses mainly the diaphragm and vertical expansion of the thoracic cavity is known as *abdominal breathing*.

As Type A is prone to thoracic breathing and Type P is prone to abdominal breathing, it is easy to identify such different interconnections between the postures and breathing patterns.

Postures and breathing are like two sides of a coin joined together as one. Combining postures and breathing will therefore achieve the best results in the correction process.

So, how can we achieve balanced breathing without being inclined to either thoracic breathing or abdominal breathing, while engaging the intercostal muscles and diaphragm together in a collaborative manner?

Axial Extension Movements for Balancing Between Spine Extension and Flexion

Performing asana in yoga is not simply about extending the spine during inhalation and flexing the spine during exhalation.

In fact, the spine is extended during inhalation, which is enabled by the expansion of the rib cage, resulting from the extension of the lumbar curve. However, because of the shortened muscles on the back, there is a limit to the expansion of the back side of the rib cage.

In order to expand the thoracic cavity fully, the ribs located in both the chest and the back regions have to expand as well. All along the sides, the front, and the back of the torso should therefore be evenly expanded, instead of just expanding at the front and contracting at the back.

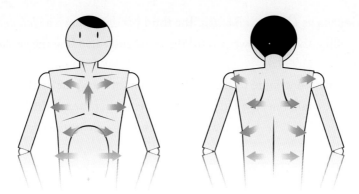

Figure 10.5. *Optimal breathing pattern.*

In this case, what should one do in order to expand the rib cage evenly in all directions when the leading pattern is thoracic breathing? Note that thoracic breathing, which uses mainly the intercostal muscles, is easy for those with excessive lumbar extension conditions. Furthermore, in this scenario, to provide an adequately strong exhalation, the abdominal muscles are activated, along with the action of drawing the tailbone down. Usually, when the exhalation stops, the inhalation takes over far too rapidly, accompanied by a raising of the tailbone and an extension of the lumbar spine.

Instead of raising the tailbone rapidly, contract the abdomen while maintaining the position of the tailbone. Slow breaths will enable elongation or axial extension of the spine, instead of extension of the lumbar spine.

As a result, not only will the ribs be evenly expanded in the front, back, left, and right, but the lower and upper parts of the thoracic cavity will be expanded as well. When such complete and balanced breathing occurs, both the diaphragm and the intercostal muscles are working simultaneously.

In the yoga tradition, a spinal control method known as *bandha* is used for axial extension of the spine. First of all, roll in the tailbone slightly and contract the lower abdomen, then draw the sit bones together while exhaling deeply. This is known as *Mula Bandha*. Then, activate the transversus abdominis muscles with the help of the rectus abdominis muscles. Relax the rectus abdominis muscles when inhalation kicks in after exhalation ends, and maintain the pressure on the lower abdomen using the transversus abdominis muscles. While doing so, the diaphragm and intercostal muscles are activated, and this is known as *Uddiyana Bandha*. The third bandha, known as *Jalandhara Bandha*, is formed by pulling the chin down toward the chest and extending the cervical vertebrae.

All three bandhas contribute to the axial extension of the spine, with the Mula Bandha taking care of the tailbone, the Uddiyana Bandha taking care of the lumbar and thoracic vertebrae, and the Jalandhara Bandha taking care of the cervical vertebrae.

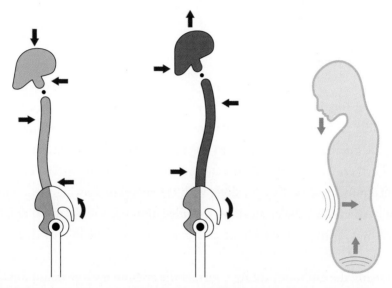

Figure 10.6. *Neutral pelvis and axial extension created by three types of bandha.*

The combined movement of breathing and postures is a technique which forms the essence of bandha; it can be used continuously, not only in still meditation poses but also in the dynamic transition of yoga asana practice.

From the Low plank pose featured in Figure 10.7, transition into positions B and C (Figures 10.8 and 10.9) continuously while exhaling deeply. Inhale slowly while transiting from position C (Figure 10.9) to position D (Figure 10.10), and extend and elongate the spine.

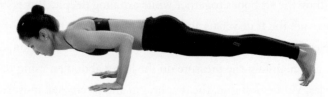

Figure 10.7. *Low plank post: position A. Focus on Mula Bandha.*

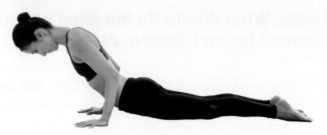

Figure 10.8. *Transition: position B. Focus on Uddiyana Bandha.*

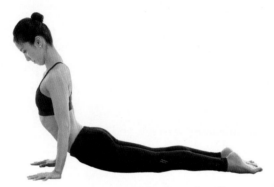

Figure 10.9. *Transition: position C. Focus on Jalandhara Bandha.*

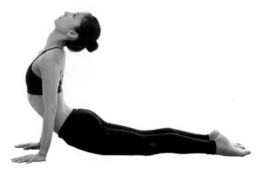

Figure 10.10. *Upward dog: position D.*

Figures 10.7, 10.8, and 10.9 demonstrate the application of Mula Bandha, Uddiyana Bandha, and Jalandhara Bandha respectively. These three bandhas are applied during the transitions between yoga poses.

Q12 Lastly, What Would Be the Most Important Element for an Effective Adjustment?

Understanding the purpose of the correction. For the effective adjustment of a posture, a prerequisite is that both the trainer and the practitioner understand the purpose behind each correction. A *correction purpose* refers to the corrective direction and the scope of correction.

If the purpose of the correction can be understood correctly, the trainer and practitioner will be working together effectively in the same corrective direction. If the correction purpose is misunderstood, however, there is the possibility of conflict between the trainer's intention and the current state of the practitioner's imbalance.

This conflict will only lead to energy wastage, and no results will be achieved. On top of that, pain or injury might also arise. Eventually, this may result in a worsening of the unbalanced condition.

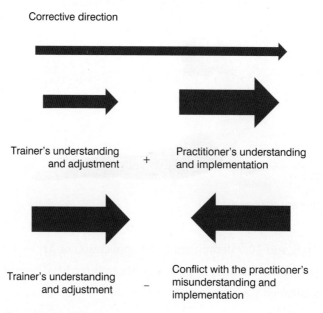

Corrective direction

Trainer's understanding and adjustment + Practitioner's understanding and implementation

Trainer's understanding and adjustment − Conflict with the practitioner's misunderstanding and implementation

Figure 10.11. *Direction of correction.*

For correct understanding and effective correction in both practice and guidance, open communication and continuous study are definite prerequisites.

Appendix

• • • • • •

Methods for Defining Body Type

Comparative Voting Method in a Small Group

Test method: voting in a small group.
Principles of test method: mutual comparison check.

Generally, there are two ways to define one's body type: subjective and objective.

The *subjective* approach enables a practitioner to recognize their own imbalances by feeling their own postures and movements.

The *objective* method consists of pinpointing one's imbalances through the help of a third party, acting as an observer; for example, section imbalances, as well as imbalances in joint movements, are identified through the eyes of a teacher. In the case of a single observer, however, the observation is based on only one person's subjective judgment and, hence, lacks the required objectivity.

In order to corroborate the objective element in the observation, the number of observers can be increased, and throughout the process, the roles of the **observers** and the **observed** are interchanged. All participants can compare the degree of imbalance in the same body type of the various **observed**, through watching them in various yoga poses.

The main advantage of a small group voting method is an increased level of understanding of the postural patterns by the participants, who embark on the collaborative process of comparison and selection.

Through participation and selection, one's incorrect perception of a body type can be corrected. Various perceptions of the unbalanced body types can be combined, compared, evaluated, discussed, and eventually made objective and scientifically validated.

SMALL GROUP VOTING ON BODY TYPE

Date: _____

Group: _____

Name								
A								
P								
C								
N								

- Group size: 6–8 members. If there are 40 participants, for example, group them into five groups of eight participants each.
- Select a facilitator within each group for a smooth operation of the session.
- The following pages present 15 different yoga poses performed by four different body types. One person is to perform all of the 15 yoga poses. Once completed, the observers are to vote on the body type (A, P, C, N) and the facilitator is to record the votes.
- Every participant will take turns performing the 15 yoga poses for the remaining participants within the group to observe and vote.

Comparison of Four Different Body Types in 15 Different Yoga Poses

1. Mountain Pose (Samasthiti)

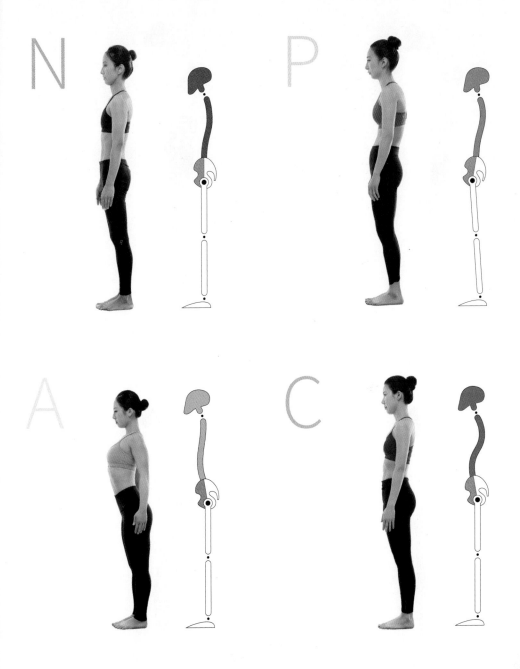

2. Hands-up Pose (Hasta Uttanasana)

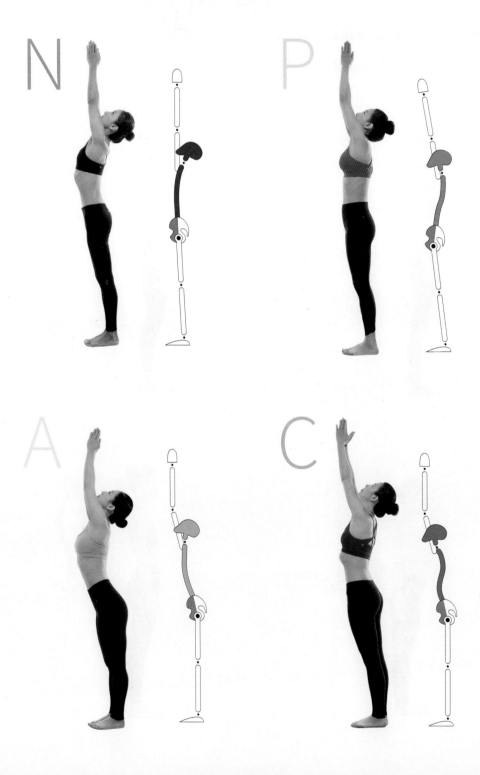

3. Standing Forward Bend Pose (Uttanasana)

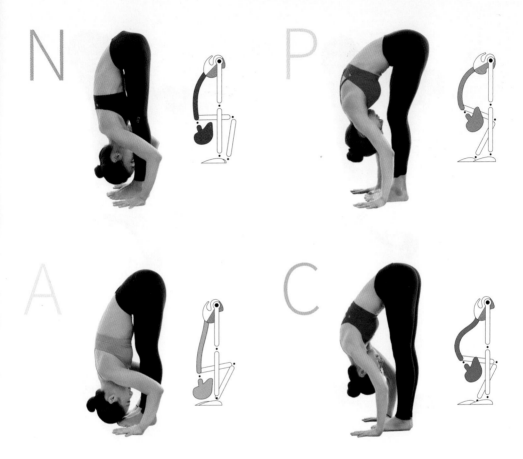

4. Standing Half Forward Bend Pose (Ardha Uttanasana)

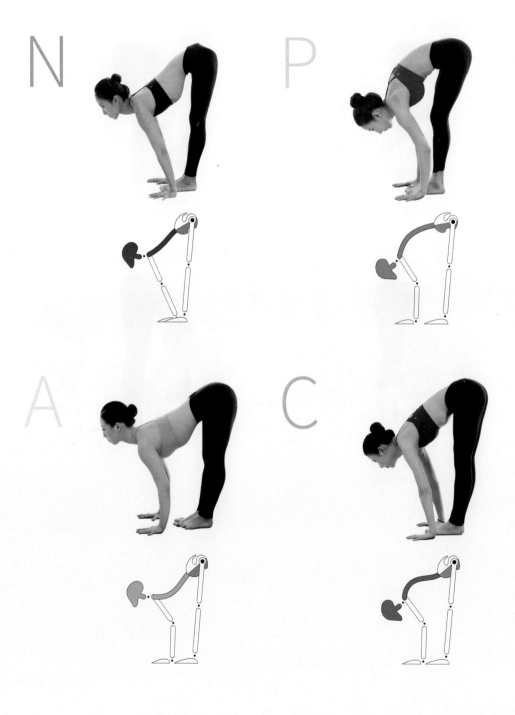

5. Plank Pose (Chaturanga Dandasana)

N

A

P

C

6. Upward-facing Dog Pose (Urdhva Mukha Svanasana)

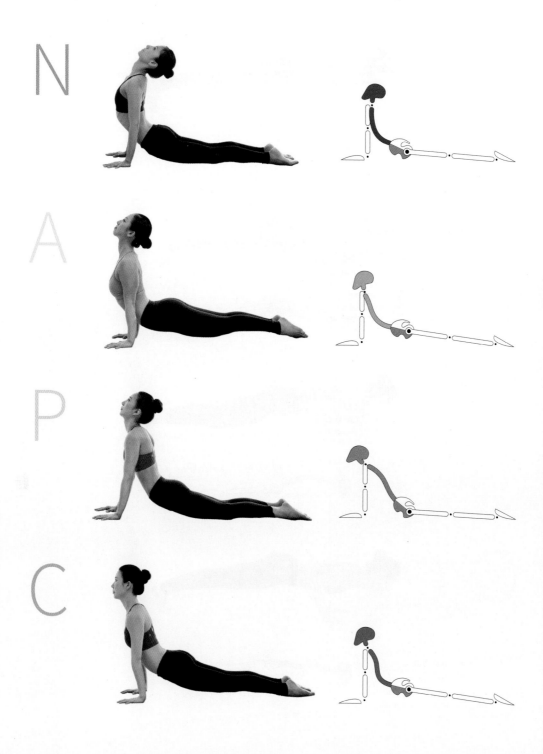

7. Downward-facing Dog Pose (Adho Mukha Svanasana)

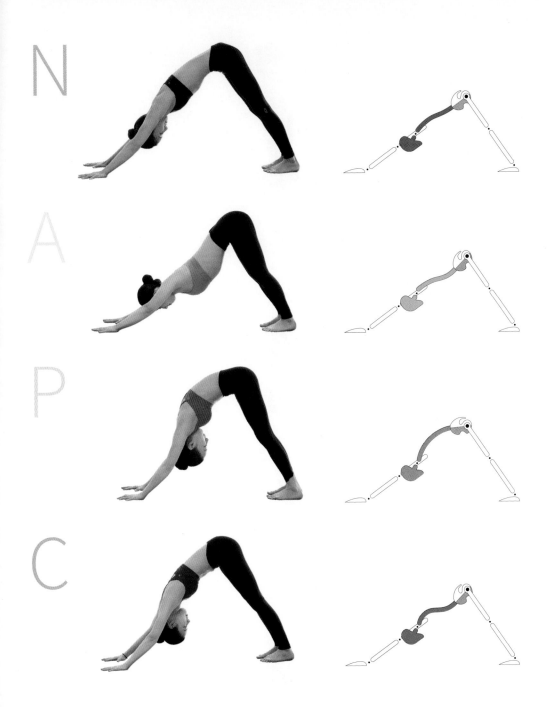

8. Staff Pose (Dandasana)

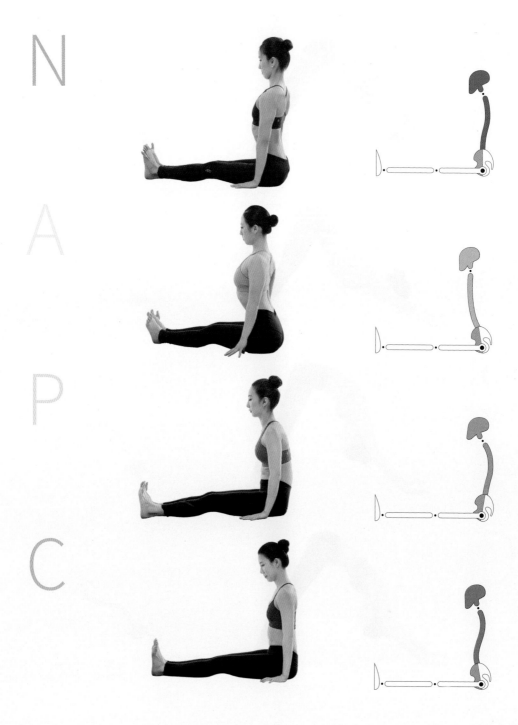

9. Seated Forward Bend Pose (Paschimottanasana)

N
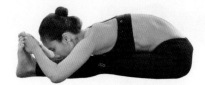
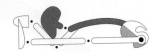

A
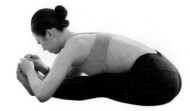
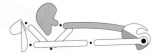

P
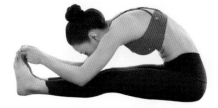
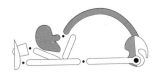

C
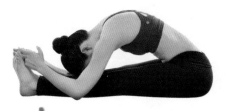
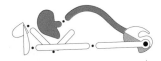

10. Upward Plank Pose (Purvottanasana)

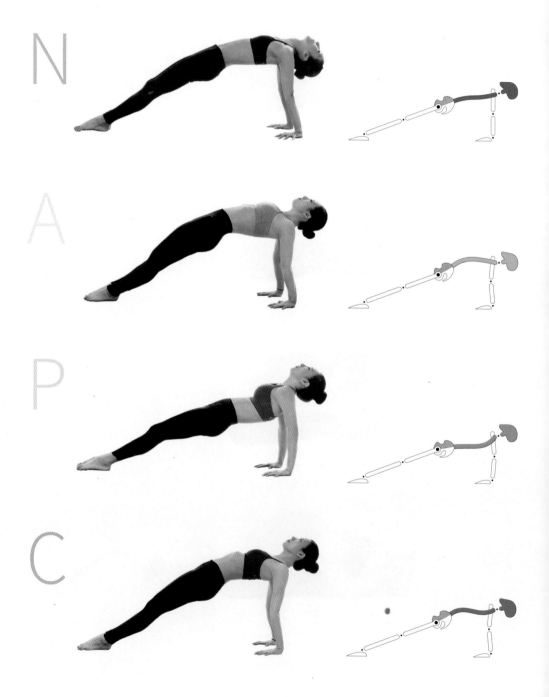

11. Bound Angle Pose A (Baddha Konasana A)

N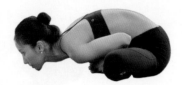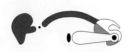

A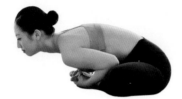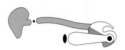

P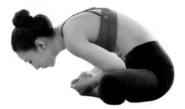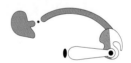

C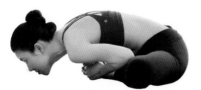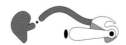

12. Bound Angle Pose B (Baddha Konasana B)

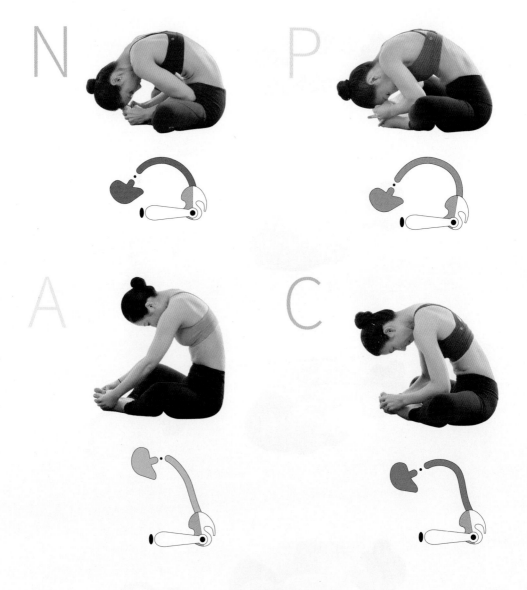

13. Sage Marichi Pose A (Marichyasana A)

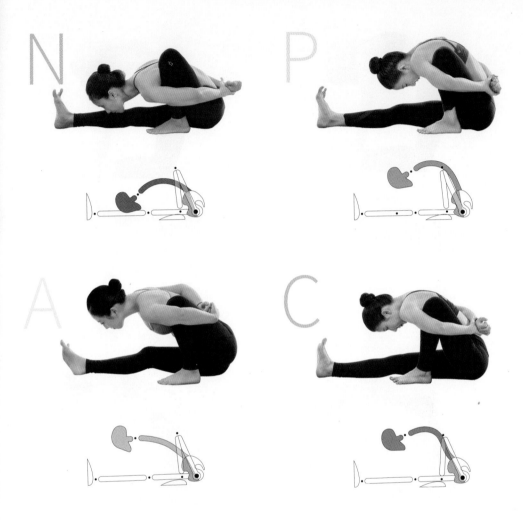

14. Camel Pose (Ustrasana)

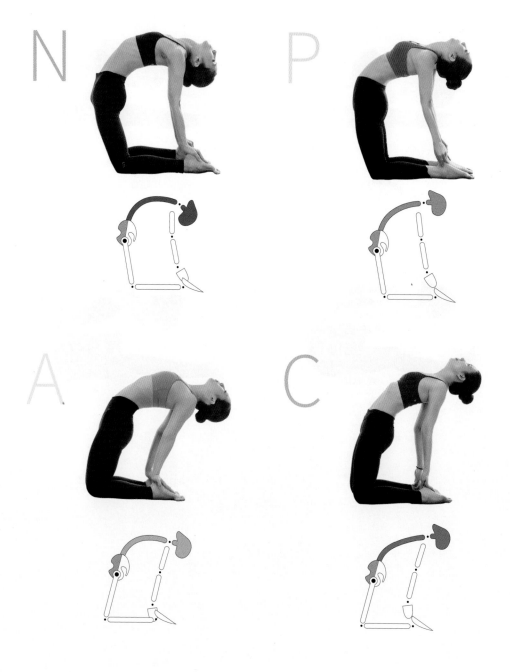

15. Backward Bending or Upward Bow Pose (Urdhva Dhanurasana)

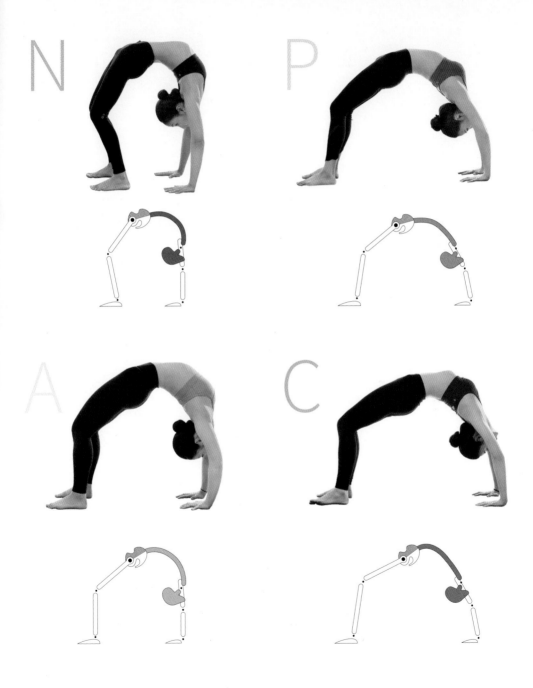

Index

About the Author

Vayu Jung Doohwa

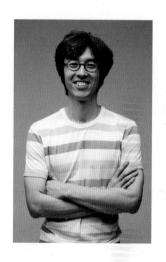

Born in 1968 in Busan, South Korea, Vayu has been fascinated by the various facets of life from an early age. His childhood was guided by his grandfather, a Confucian scholar; the passing of his grandfather made Vayu truly enquire into the fundamental questions of life: "Who am I?"; "Where am I from?"; "What is the purpose of life?". Longing for answers, at the age of fifteen Vayu began a period of intensive meditation with a Zen master at a Buddhist temple.

In his mid-twenties, to support himself and his family, Vayu completed a university degree in pharmacy, and opened his own pharmacy in Seoul. His spiritual search and questioning, however, never ceased. In 1996 Vayu embarked on his yoga journey, paying his first visit to India in 2001, while researching the roots of yoga. Eventually, from 2005 to 2007, he discovered the Ashtanga Yoga tradition, which he felt a connection with, practicing with Guruji Sri K. Pattabhi Jois.

In 2008 Vayu met John Scott in Beijing; this encounter led Vayu to realize the true meaning of Vinyasa. The meeting with his new-found teacher was followed by his translating of John Scott's book *Ashtanga Yoga* into Korean, and subsequently several years of studying with John on the Teacher Training Course at Stillpoint Yoga in New Zealand.

Vayu started teaching traditional Mysore-style yoga classes in his hometown of Busan in 2007, and he established the Yoga VnA studio in 2010. Since then he has been working on the contemporary scientific interpretations of the traditional Ashtanga yoga.

Vayu has held more than 100 yoga anatomy workshops in Korea and China. He is a leader of the faculty of anatomy at Yoga VnA and Yoga Kula in Korea and the John Scott Yoga China Teacher Training Course. He published his first book, *The Art of Observing and Adjusting: An Innovative Guide to Yoga Asana Adjustment for Your Postural Type* in Korean in 2016, and successfully presented the concepts of the book at the teachers' workshop of John Scott Yoga in London. Vayu is currently working on his second book, about yoga adjustments for symmetric imbalance.